A Factual Guide by the

World's Leading Clinical Expert

MORGELLONS:

THE LEGITIMIZATION

OF A DISEASE

Dr. Ginger Savely

Library of Congress Cataloging-in-Publication Data is available on file.

In an effort to keep sales prices down, this book has been printed in black and white. Please visit www.gingersavely.com/morgellons-book **to access color versions of all photographs.**

Cover design by Ruben de Haas
Cover photo credit Denise Moudree

ISBN
E-Book: 978-0-9979200-0-0
Paperback: 978-0-9979200-2-4

Printed in the United States of America

DEDICATION

Travis Wilson was one of many "orphan patients" abandoned by the health care system because he did not have the good fortune to contract a known and socially accepted disease. To Travis, for the loss of his young life, and to the many other Morgellons patients who have suffered in isolation and fear, I dedicate this work.

FOREWORD

There is a rapidly growing interest in Morgellons disease as evidenced by the fact that research papers on the topic have been among the most highly accessed scientific research on the Internet for the past few years. As director of the Charles E. Holman Morgellons Disease Foundation (CEHMDF), I hear from 5 to 10 new patients daily who have symptoms consistent with the disease and who have hit brick walls trying to access medical care.

In our early years, the CEHMDF would field calls from hostile doctors, disgruntled that we were validating the symptoms reported by Morgellons patients. Today we hear more often from doctors who are baffled and at a loss to know what to do for the patients presenting to their practices with the debilitating symptoms of this new and misunderstood disease. As more and more research is published in the medical literature, Morgellons disease is slowly gaining acceptance as an infectious disease despite an unusually fierce opposition that strives to keep it tucked away and dismissed as purely psychiatric in origin.

Dr. Ginger Savely was the first pioneering medical provider to take her Morgellons patients' symptoms seriously and work to legitimize the disease. She took on this very challenging patient population and stood by them in their darkest hours. Dr. Savely listened to her patients and looked at the blatant objective evidence. She was the first to speak out publicly about this serious health crisis and she has continued throughout the years to stand up for the reality of Morgellons disease through her numerous published articles, interviews, and presentations at medical conferences. Dr. Savely has been a lifeline for hundreds of suffering people who have lost their way and given up hope of ever receiving medical attention for their unusual and agonizing symptoms. She has worked to educate her peers and has been committed to helping her patients.

At a time when interest in Morgellons disease is at an all time high, this detailed first-hand account of the Morgellons journey is a much-needed resource. With clarity, personal style and years of experience, Dr. Savely has taken on a challenging and highly controversial subject. Using up-to-the-minute scientific findings, color photographs and sweeping examples she has illuminated the path to recognition of this debilitating and disfiguring disease, previously orphaned by the medical community.

We have come a long way against great odds on our journey to legitimize Morgellons disease. Dr. Savely paved the earliest path on the rockiest road to make this progress possible. I have no doubt that Morgellons disease will eventually be fully recognized worldwide by health agencies and the medical community at large because the scientific evidence has reached an undeniable point. I firmly believe that in time the truth will prevail.

This book provides long-awaited answers to the vital questions being posed by thousands of patients and clinicians about this unthinkable disease. In reading Dr. Savely's poignant narrative, you will learn to separate fact from myth and rumor from reality. This book will be a valuable resource for Morgellons patients and their families and friends and will serve as a guide for clinicians who are open-minded and committed to the health of their patients.

Cindy Casey-Holman, RN
Director, The Charles E. Holman Morgellons
Disease Foundation www.MorgellonsDisease.org

"Never doubt that a small group of thoughtful, committed citizens can change the world; indeed it's the only thing that ever has."

— Margaret Mead

INTRODUCTION

In 2003 I was working as a primary care nurse practitioner in a family practice clinic in Austin, Texas. A few years earlier I had become interested in treating Lyme disease after my teenage daughter became very ill with it. Lyme disease, a tickborne infection caused by the bacteria *Borrelia burgdorferi*, is most commonly seen in the northeastern United States but cases have been reported in all 50 states. By 2003 about 30% of my patients were Lyme disease patients because as I became more interested and knowledgeable about the disease, people who suspected that they had it began to seek me out.

One of my Lyme disease patients had previously been diagnosed with ALS (amyotrophic lateral sclerosis), a progressive and fatal neurodegenerative disease involving gradual atrophy of muscles of the body. When he first became ill he had been an active young man who led hikes through the mountains in Colorado. By the time I saw him he was expected to live no longer than another year. I began treating him with antibiotics after discovering that his Lyme Western Blot blood test was positive. Almost miraculously, he slowly began to improve.

Jim Bergamo, a news reporter with an Austin TV station, caught wind of the story of this young man who was improving from an incurable condition, and thought it would make a compelling human-interest story for the evening news. He and his crew came to my office and taped a TV news segment about this ALS patient, his illness and my treatment of him. As Jim left the office and thanked me for the story I said, "If you think this was interesting you've GOT to come back and do a story on Morgellons disease!"

Of course, I had to explain what I meant by this because at that point no one had heard of Morgellons (pronounced with a soft G) disease. I explained that a dozen or so of my Lyme patients had mysterious, spontaneously appearing, slow-healing lesions with unusual colored filaments embedded in and/or extruding from their skin. Other doctors had diagnosed these patients with "Delusions of Parasitosis" but I was beginning to have some success treating them with antibiotics. Their symptoms were varied, unexplainable and bizarre. I knew these patients were not delusional because I had observed the filaments myself using lighted magnification. I had tried to extract the embedded filaments but since they were firmly and deeply attached my attempts to remove them caused patients deep, radiating pain.

I had learned from my colleague William Harvey, M.D. of Houston, TX (now deceased) that there was a name for the filament condition – Morgellons disease. The name was given by a microbiologist in Pennsylvania whose 3-year-old son had the symptoms. So, Jim Bergamo and his team returned once more to my office to make what was to become a powerful, award-winning news segment about Morgellons disease. The day after the segment aired, dozens of people began calling my office, excited to know that there were other people with their unusual symptoms and that there was actually a name for their condition.

That was the start of an influx of patients with the unusual symptoms of Morgellons disease. What impressed me right away was that all of these people described the EXACT same long list of perplexing symptoms. This was before the disease had developed media notoriety so patients could not have been telling me the "right" symptoms in order to gain my attention. In fact, these patients were often hard-working West Texas ranchers who certainly didn't have hypochondriacal tendencies or a habit of surfing the net to find the disease du jour, as was being suggested by the naysayers in the medical establishment.

At first, I panicked. I was not an expert on this disease (not that anyone was) and I had no idea what I was going to do with all of these people. Since I had first noted the symptoms in a subset of my Lyme disease patients I decided that the first thing I would do would be to test these filament disease patients for Lyme disease. So, I began ordering blood tests to look for Lyme and other tickborne diseases and almost all of the Morgellons patients were positive for at least one of the tickborne infections. With antibiotic treatment, they began to improve. They came from all walks of life, from all over the state of Texas, neighboring states and even California. There were ranch hands from west Texas, landscapers, attorneys, physicians, nurses, secretaries, carpenters and college professors. Every career, race, age and socio-economic group was represented.

Then the barrage of publicity began. About 10 years ago, Morgellons disease enjoyed a brief flurry of notoriety when the media first became aware of its attention-grabbing salability. I published numerous journal articles and was interviewed for articles in *The Washington Post,*

San Francisco Chronicle, Los Angeles Times, and *Dallas Observer*. Magazines such as *Psychology Today, The Texas Monthly* and *Popular Mechanics* published articles on the topic and radio and television interviews I gave were played extensively on affiliated networks. One of my patients and I were featured in a segment of the Animal Planet series, *Monsters Inside Me*, as well as an episode of Discovery Heath Channel's *Mystery ER.* A taped interview of us was shown on the *Rachel Ray Show*.

In 2006, my work was featured in a 6-minute segment taped for the *Diane Rehm Show*. When the network's crew arrived to spend 3 days taping in my San Francisco office, it was clear from the looks on their faces and their tones of voice that they were highly skeptical and expected to produce a segment about people with delusions. By the time they left to fly back to New York City they were believers – they could not deny the existence of MD after what they had observed.

I naively assumed that dermatologists around the world would be very excited about this new Morgellons disease. I thought they would be fascinated and intrigued to learn about a novel skin condition, which would presumably offer a welcome relief from the monotony of treating teenaged acne. I could not have been more mistaken. Instead of being captivated by the uniqueness of the disease, dermatologists would refer patients to psychiatrists without even examining the skin or asking further questions of the patients. Intellectual curiosity, I soon learned, is no longer a strong suit of the majority of those practicing medicine.

I was harshly criticized by my colleagues who accused me of "playing into" the psychosis of these patients by diagnosing them with a medical condition and treating them with antibiotics. It did not matter that patients were getting better – my critics claimed this was probably a placebo reaction to patients being heard and validated.

Meanwhile, there still remained the baffling questions: what was causing these unusual symptoms and why did some patients respond better to treatment than others? In fact, as time went on it became clear that many did not respond to Lyme disease treatment, resulting in my early experimentation with other anti-infective medications such as anthelminthics, antiparasitics, antifungals, antivirals and many different types of antibiotics, hoping to discover the perfect medication cocktail to deliver these poor souls from their misery. But, without knowledge of the causative pathogen, I was flying on a wing and a prayer.

This book is a result of my experience treating hundreds of Morgellons patients for over a decade. Most of what I chronicle here is based on personal clinical experience. At one point 80% of my practice was devoted to treating Morgellons disease. I have learned through trial and error but mostly through the feedback of my courageous patients. Far from being a group of "crazy people" (as most of the medical world has labeled them), I have found my patients with Morgellons disease to be good-willed, sane, brave, hard-working people, trying to make the best of a horrific situation. I thank them all for willingly becoming "lab rats" in an ongoing treatment experiment. I will forever be humbled by their strength and perseverance and honored by their trust and faith in me.

TABLE OF CONTENTS

Part One

Truth is Stranger then Fiction

"All truth passes through three stages. First, it is ridiculed. Second, it is violently opposed. Third, it is accepted as being self-evident".

— Arthur Schopenhauer

CINDY'S STORY

"Oh, my gosh…. that is so bizarre!" "What could possibly cause that?" "Have you seen a dermatologist?" "What are you going to do?" A group of nurses gathers around the nurse's station examining their co-worker's arms. They are intrigued yet somewhat frightened by the unusual skin condition that is causing their friend's skin to erupt and produce brightly colored filaments.

A 60x-powered, hand-held lighted magnifier enables the nurses to see the unusual filaments that are intertwined in masses beneath their co-worker's skin. One of the nurses motions for the doctor on call to come and take a look. It is not unusual at this teaching hospital for staff to gather to assess a patient with an unusual condition, learn about a new monitoring device, or brainstorm about a problematic wound. But what is unusual this time is that the patient is one of their own, a respected and experienced member of the team.

No Help From the Dermatologists

Cindy Casey, RN had worked as a staff nurse and charge nurse in this Medical Specialty Intensive Care Unit for over 15 years. She had already seen four dermatologists for her peculiar symptoms and none of them was even willing to look at the filaments she described. She was hastily dismissed as delusional or self-mutilating and was offered no more than antipsychotics. Despite her disfiguring lesions and debilitating symptoms, Cindy was released to continue working in her job as staff nurse/relief charge nurse in a 21-bed critical care unit.

The lesions continued to appear spontaneously and the symptoms intensified. The itching and crawling sensations became unbearable and soon Cindy's entire body was covered with painful, oozing, disfiguring lesions. Various antihistamines and medications for neuropathies were all ineffective in controlling the insatiable itch and crawling sensations. Black specks and bizarre filaments in white, clear, black, red, and blue emerged from unbroken skin and the edges of the open lesions turned black. Cindy's co-workers, friends, and family could see these strange exudates with their own eyes. They knew Cindy as a calm, competent, and well-adjusted woman and certainly not delusional.

The 5th dermatologist Cindy consulted took her seriously enough to conduct a thorough medical workup including comprehensive blood work, chest x-ray, a series of stool specimens and referral to a neurologist to rule out neuropathy as a cause of the unusual sensations. Yet even this dermatologist had no interest in looking carefully at the microscopic debris that was torturing Cindy day and night. Cindy could only guess that the doctor's reluctance to examine her skin had something to do with not wanting to encourage her "delusion". A skin biopsy was performed at Cindy's insistence but the report described the filaments as textile contaminants. All test results were normal and again, there were no answers.

When In Doubt, Diagnose a Psychiatric Condition?

Cindy continued working and was very open about her illness with her colleagues. Her nurse manager became concerned that Cindy's condition might be contagious, putting the hospital unit's immune-compromised patients at risk. Furthermore, the open lesions that Cindy was unable to occlude would put her at risk for hospital-acquired infections. Cindy's nurse manager consulted the infectious disease specialists in the unit for advice. Initially, these specialists seemed concerned but after making a call to Cindy's dermatologist, they too suspected her problems were psychiatric in origin.

The last dermatologist and his residents had alluded to a possible psychological origin of Cindy's illness but had never come out and said anything definitive. When Cindy's husband Charles asked directly for a diagnosis, the residents became uneasy and evasive. Charles asked again and was told: "It is known as different things in different countries". Charles replied with "Okay…. so let's start with what it is referred to in the United States". In a meek voice and without making eye contact, one of the residents reluctantly replied "Delusions of Parasitosis."

Delusions of Parasitosis

Delusions of Parasitosis (DOP), also known as Delusional Parasitosis or Ekbom's Syndrome, is a psychiatric disorder in which patients mistakenly believe they are infested with parasites. In medical school physicians learn of the "matchbox sign" of DOP, so named because in earlier times patients would present the debris from their lesions in a matchbox. DOP is actually very rare and oddly those diagnosed with it have no prior history of mental illness. In fact, patients seem cognitively intact in every way while insistent that there is something inside of them causing itching and other disturbing sensations. Some of the earliest patients with these symptoms expressed the belief that their symptoms were due to a parasite.

However, because a known parasite could not be identified on a superficial exam, doctors assumed that the patients were imagining things.

In Search of Answers

Cindy and Charles were stunned by the DOP diagnosis. Cindy had never mentioned parasites nor did she have a belief that parasites were the cause of her problems. She had no personal or family history of mental disorders and in fact, she was a newlywed and the happiest she had been in her life. If the doctors believed she had a psychiatric problem, why had they not referred her to a psychiatrist? Charles asked the dermatologist for treatment recommendations. His reply was: "There is nothing we can do for the condition of her skin. We can only offer medications that may help her to perceive her skin differently." Unfortunately, the prescribed medications caused incapacitating sedation and the horrifying symptoms remained unchanged.

Refusing to accept the DOP diagnosis, Cindy and Charles continued to search for an explanation for Cindy's frightening and debilitating symptoms. Charles created a website and began maintaining a blog detailing the trials and tribulations of their quest. When they first heard the term Morgellons disease (MD), found out there was a website and realized that Cindy had the characteristic symptoms, they had their first glimmer of hope. At least Cindy was not alone and if there were others afflicted with her condition, surely help would follow. But finding a name for Cindy's condition and knowing that there were others in her situation were only the first steps in what was to become a frustrating and wearisome journey. Few healthcare providers were willing to even admit the disease was real, much less try to help the patients who were suffering from it.

Cindy started granting interviews for television and newspapers regarding her mysterious illness. After her first appearance on

TV, Cindy began hearing from patients all over the United States. It was then that she knew she had done the right thing by going public with her symptoms. At the same time, she realized that her life would never be the same.

The Charles E. Holman Foundation

Cindy worked her last shift as a nurse in November 2005. She misses her job and the people she worked with for 16 years. Although she has improved considerably by taking antibiotics, Cindy still struggles with Morgellons symptoms daily and her disfigured body bears little resemblance to the vibrant, healthy nurse that she once was. She now lives on Social Security Disability Insurance and has become a passionate advocate for Morgellons patients all over the world. In 2007 Cindy started a non-profit foundation named *The Charles E. Holman Morgellons Disease Foundation* (CEHMDF) in honor of the husband she had just lost to an untimely death. Charles had seen Cindy through her most difficult times and she still feels fortunate that she had his support as well as that of her family and friends who took her symptoms seriously from the beginning. Since its inception, the CEHMDF has worked tirelessly to raise awareness of the disease and has held an annual conference in Austin, Texas for health care providers and patients to network, learn new research findings and share theories of etiology and treatment strategies.

As the CEHMDF continues to educate health care providers about MD. most are surprised to learn that the disease is not a new phenomenon. It has only recently gained media notoriety but some version of the disease has been around a long time. In the next chapter, I will review what we know about the history of this bizarre disease.

MORGELLONS: NOT A NEW DISEASE

A 17th-century British physician, Sir Thomas Browne, was the first to describe a disease resembling what we currently think of as Morgellons disease. Browne was a veritable Renaissance man with interest and expertise in history, philosophy, religion, linguistics and pathology. In a 1674 letter to a friend, Browne wrote the following perplexing passage, referring to a time when he was a medical student in France:

> *"Hairs which have most amused me have not been in the face or head, but on the Back, and not in Men but Children, as I long ago observed in that endemial Distemper of little Children in Languedock, called the Morgellons, wherein they critically break out with harsh Hairs on their Backs, which takes off the unquiet symptoms of the Disease, and delivers them from Coughs and Convulsions".*

The condition had been known as *pilaris affectio* ("hair affection") by physicians as far back as 1544 and was associated with pain, itching, convulsions, and wasting in its young victims. In some writings, the "hairs" were referred to as "little worms with black heads."

Why Browne referred to the condition as "the Morgellons" in his writings is not clear, although it may have been his English derivation of the term "Mousquelons", meaning the tiny hook at the end of a spindle, and the French provincial name for the disease in the 17th century. But, C.E. Kellett, MD (1908-78), pediatrician and owner of a collection of books and essays on 16th and 17th-century European medicine, postulated that the word may have derived from the Provincial word "muscula", a tiny fly.

Although similarities exist between the disease currently known as Morgellons and the disease described in the 17th century, the old illustrations do not exactly match what is seen today. Moreover, the modern day illness is seen in adults as well as children and convulsions are not reported as one of the symptoms.

Dr. Michele Ettmuller's 1682 microscopic drawings of objects associated with what was then believed to be a worm infestation of children appear somewhat similar to microscopic views of filaments from present-day sufferers of MD. Ettmuller's drawings exhibit a long narrow segmented filament with a bulbous end, from which emanate little hooks and hairs (see picture on next page). Morgellons patients often describe a similar appearance of the filaments that exit their lesions but none of us who have been treating these patients or researching their condition have seen anything that exactly matches Ettmuller's drawings.

In the June 22, 1946 edition of the *British Medical Journal*, a letter to the editor entitled *"Myasis, 'Fillan' and 'The Morgellons' "* was written by A.H. Emslie-Smith, a microbiologist with the Royal Army Medical Corps and the department of bacteriology at King's College, Newcastle upon Tyne. Smith proposed that what had previously been known as Morgellons disease may have actually been an infestation by larvae of the cattle pest, *Hypoderma bovis* (gadfly), working their way through the skin. We now know that this is not the case.

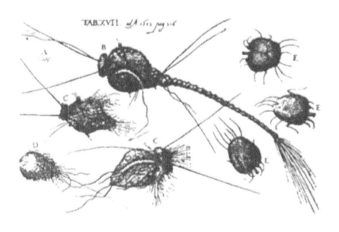

Morgellons disease was not mentioned again until Mary Leitao brought it to modern day attention in 2001. A microbiology-trained mother of three, living in Pennsylvania, Leitao noted a non-healing lesion on the lower lip of her young son. The child complained that there were "bugs"

under his skin and when Leitao looked at a scab from his lesion under magnification she noted deeply embedded blue and red filaments that fluoresced under ultraviolet light.

Unable to find answers for her son's perplexing condition from the physicians she consulted, Leitao, like many others who are faced with unidentifiable diseases, began scouring the Internet for answers. When she uncovered Dr. Thomas Browne's writings she thought that his 17th-century description sounded similar to what was happening to her young son. In 2002, Leitao re-birthed the name Morgellons disease (MD) to describe her son's ailment and proceeded to found a not-for-profit organization named The Morgellons Research Foundation (MRF) with the goal of garnering serious attention for the disease. The website included a database where patients could report their symptoms.

The organization's website began to disseminate information and ask those with MD symptoms to come forward and be counted. By 2009 the number of self-reported cases exceeded 14,000 with the tally rapidly increasing daily. The original focus was on skin symptoms but soon other symptoms within the patient group became recognized, such as disabling fatigue, life-altering cognitive decline, musculoskeletal pain, and mood disorders. Leitao's website and the original MRF became inactive in early 2012 and the website domain name was taken over by promoters of the chemtrail theory of Morgellons (more about this later). Those who search for the MRF website these days are <u>not</u> seeing the website originally founded by Mary Leitao.

My suspicion is that Morgellons disease goes back many centuries, probably even before the mention of it by Sir Thomas Browne in the 17th century. During the 19th and 20th centuries patient complaints of crawling sensations and filaments resulted in a delusional diagnosis because it was believed that patients were imagining bugs crawling on them and that the filaments and other debris from their skin were environmental contaminants. By the 21st century, patients learned to keep quiet about their symptoms for fear of being diagnosed psychotic, ruining their chances of a respectable job and place in society. The disease did not decrease in incidence; people just did not want to deal with the negative reactions to their complaints.

One of my MD patients symptoms date back to 1954 – you will read his story in the next chapter. Thus, there are reasons to believe that Morgellons disease is not new to this century or even to the last. What has changed is awareness, thanks to the rapid spread of information through the Internet, enabling thousands of people to come out of the shadows and be validated. Morgellons patients, who have suffered for more than 15 years, before a name was given for their condition or their disease was discussed in the media, have experienced the worst isolation and prejudicial treatment. Bill Pitt was one such patient.

WHEN NOTHING SEEMS RIGHT, CRAZY MAKES SENSE

"Poster boy for Morgellons disease". That is what I used to call him. He grinned and bore the title proudly. None of the patients I have treated for Morgellons disease have suffered as long as Bill Pitt did. He first came to my San Francisco office in 2005, a tall, good-looking man with a booming laugh and language that would make a sailor blush. Bill was big and tough and street smart but underneath his bulletproof exterior was a thoughtful, intelligent and sensitive soul.

It was impossible not to love Bill and all of us in the office did. He was a character, that's for sure. He made us laugh with his sarcastic wit and brought tears to our eyes with his honest, self-deprecating insights. Not surprisingly, there was anger and resentment beneath his jovial exterior and at times it would break through as he recounted the many years of suffering he had endured due to a medical establishment unwilling to open their eyes to the strange malady that plagued him.

He used to call me "Dr. Doll". Others might have seen this as chauvinistic but I didn't take it that way. He was always appropriate with me and I knew it was his tender way of showing me respect. He worried about me constantly. He was afraid that by helping bring MD to the public eye I had put myself at some kind of risk. He told me not to drive on back roads alone. (He saw me as another Erin Brockovich and feared I would meet her same fate.) At the 5-year anniversary of our doctor/patient relationship Bill sent me a gift – a beautiful slice of petrified wood. He had searched online and discovered that 5 years is the wooden anniversary. He was known for sweet gestures like this.

Despite what you will read in his personal account that follows, Bill not only considered suicide but attempted it on several occasions. Each time that a suicide attempt failed he would joke and say that he was not even able to do suicide right. I pointed out to him that maybe the reason he did not succeed was that his presence here on earth was essential to unlocking the key to this mysterious disease.

I urged Bill to write about his life with Morgellons disease because I felt it was vital for people to know how long its victims have been suffering in silence. Having recently learned with great sadness of Bill's passing due to natural causes, I was moved to retrieve his notes and review them. My last doctor-patient encounter with him was 2 months before his death. Re-reading his words made me sad and made me smile. I was obliged to edit his writing somewhat (punctuation was not his forte) and clean up the language here and there (he had a predilection for four letter words) but I believe his raw narrative is moving and gives insight into the isolation suffered by MD patients.

[Note: Bill chose to use the term fiber where I use the word filament. I am concerned that the word fiber is suggestive of textiles and I choose not to use terminology that promotes the continued incorrect belief that the filaments in MD patients are textile fibers. However, I want to present Bill's narrative just as he wrote it.]

Here is Bill's story in his own words:

For me, it started at an early age. I was just 6 years old in 1954 when I first noticed "things" would appear on or in my skin, disappearing as quickly as they appeared. By the age of 7, I was seeing spinning, moving hairs on my skin. My mom would yank them out when she felt I was getting too fascinated by what these "hairs" were doing. Around this same time, my father became ill with sores on his feet and legs. He spent long nights digging into his sores. He was sure that there was something deep inside of him causing his sores and his pain and he wasn't going to stop until he could remove the source of his torture. In fact, he had little time for anything else but trying to prove to himself and his doctors that something unusual was going on.

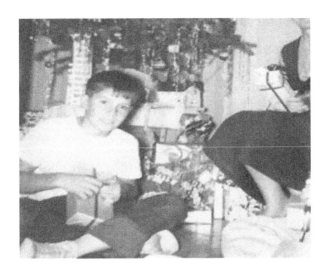

Bill, Christmas of 1958, 10 years old.

My Dad continued like this until he died when I was 12 years old. He died on the operating table at Los Angeles General Hospital when the doctors said there was nothing left to do but amputate his legs to remove the gaping sores and his tormenting belief that something was boring its way through his skin. This was the cure in 1960. The doctor that led the team on my father's case resigned shortly after Dad died and he and his family moved out of California. He was kind enough to stop by our house to say how sorry he was and that something like this should not have happened in an age of modern medicine.

I look back now and laugh. I think it was right then that I realized if I was going to survive this mystery disease I would need to rely on myself and what I knew to be the truth. I realized that I was alone in this and it seemed the world was against me. Shortly before he died my Dad told me to stay strong no matter what other people might say about our strange affliction.

So began decades of back glances, snide remarks and doctor referrals to mental heath professionals who supposedly knew what to do with "delusional" people like me. As a kid, I was in and out of a galvanized metal tub where I soaked in vinegar or baking soda or whatever other suggestion was given for my almost constant rashes. It appeared that I had allergies and everyone would call me "poor Billy, the little rash boy".

Once, when I was 11 years old, I laid on the floor of our living room crying in pain. My bones and all of my joints hurt so badly that all I was able to do was lie on the floor curled up in a ball. My mother talked with the family doctor and he thought it best that I be taken to Children's Hospital in Los Angeles. We didn't have a car so I was put in a shopping cart and wheeled to the bus stop. On the bus I lay on the floor writhing in pain. Less than half way to Children's Hospital the bus driver pulled over and called a taxi for my mom and me. He was kind enough to pay the taxi fare since we didn't have money for such things. I can remember the ride but little of anything but pain and tears after we arrived at the hospital. I was released from the hospital a day and a half later with a diagnosis of "growing pains". That was "modern medicine".

Life became more or less normal and when I got older and enlisted in the Navy in 1965 I passed all *the physicals. How could anything be wrong with me when I got a stamp of approval from the US Government? Yet, I became more cautious about what I said or did about my itching and fibers and I knew with greater intensity that something was wrong with the system. I began to think of myself as a stranger here on earth and that this disease and I shared a different reality.*

My military enlistment ended and I was now in my 20's. I was scrubbing my skin and spending hours in the water at the beach chasing these darned fibers. I spent all my free time working out, soaking in the steam room and sauna and scrubbing away at my skin. The rashes still came and went and new feelings came that made me feel as if I was being eaten alive and my body and my mind were being snatched away from me. I couldn't help but think that a new life form had taken over my body and was capable of stealing my life right in front of everyone. And I was the only person who could see it.

It was insanity. I played with that in order to survive. I hid in plain sight - sometimes I hid even from myself. I was that crazy dude with weird stories. So as I went into my 30s and 40s what I know now as Morgellons disease took me to more doctors than most people ever see in a lifetime. I even went to other countries searching out folk healers. In Mexico, they packed me in lard, coated me in flour and bathed me in milk all to draw out the "devils fingers". They were familiar with what was going on with me and told me I had "cactus man disease". And still, the rashes came.

As the fibers increased my skin became alien to me, as though I was being encased in reptilian gauze. I could have gone stark raving mad at any time but instead, I became a warrior against everything that stood in my way. Nothing was more important than giving this thing a name and finding one other person on this planet that could see and believe what I was living with. Family, friends, and anyone who dared look sideways at me I now perceived as against me. Everyone became my enemy as much as the disease inside me. Was I the harbinger of a plague that would destroy or forever change the world in some evil way? I was alone, just "Melvins" and me. That was the name I had given to my disease. I don't know why. I just needed it to have a name. It was probably my Mom who first coined the name by saying "Billy is having a Melvin fit".

For most of my life, I worked as a machinist on different railroads here in the U.S. There would be periods of being laid off and during one of those times I found work as a heavy machine operator and mechanic at a surface mine in Ventura County, CA. Just after completing a new clearing out on a high ridge it was fantastic to look out over the Pacific, the sunset casting gleaming beams into the cab of my D10 dozer.

One day at work I was bitten by some kind of bug and it stung like crazy. Within the first hour, a bull's eye rash formed on my leg [a bull's eye rash is the classic diagnostic feature of Lyme disease]. The boss sent me to an urgent care center where I was given antibiotics and told to go home, put the leg up and rest. I stayed in bed for a couple of days and the bull's eye rash turned into a festering mass of what looked like a French pastry gone mad. I called the doctor and he sent me to another doctor who said "Wow!" put me on stronger antibiotics and sent me home again. Fourteen days went by and the bull's eye rash began to disappear - until the antibiotics ran out. Then the rash came back with a vengeance.

This time, I was sent to the UCLA Medical center where I took part in a doctor's round table event. There were about 100 physicians with lots of looking and hmm'ing. Some had cameras and snapped shots with different colored backdrops to make the bull's eye rash "pop" in the photos. More antibiotics were prescribed and in the end, I was told my Lyme test was negative. It remained negative for another 10 years until I finally saw a Lyme expert and had a better test done. Of course, this delayed-diagnosis worked well for my employer because by then time had expired for me to file any type of a claim. The good news was that I was able to go back to work at my regular job and the insurance company could not write it off as a pre-existing condition. This is all interesting because it has now been seen that a large percentage of Morgellons patients have Lyme disease and co-infections, which I refer to as the "bacterial coalition". My Lyme expert told me that I had a number of different coalition bacteria working their way through my body.

During the time from the late 70s into the mid-90s I lived an almost nomadic life. My home, at first an oversized camper, later became a 36-foot 5th wheel trailer with all the amenities. I would move from spot to spot sometimes staying in hotels or nicer motels. I was buying new clothes about 5 times a week, new sheets too. Socks and underwear I just tossed in the trash. And I say I was never crazy! All I was trying to do was stay ahead of the fibers and the dirty feeling and the crawling, biting madness that stole my sleep. I lived in driveways and in back alleys. Even though I still held my job some people thought that I was a fugitive of some kind. So yes, there was *the crazy but there was a lot of comedy involved too! If you can't laugh you won't survive!*

As the 1990s rolled on I realized I needed to settle somewhere. A change in railroad jobs took me to Barstow, California of all places – Barstow, known for taking advantage of the traveler in distress. But it was also in Barstow that I met and worked with a guy who while at work one day asked if I felt OK. "Why?" I asked. "Well, because you're several different colors and it looks like s**t is coming out of your skin". Yep, he actually said that. He was right and he could see it for what it was. So things were changing - someone other than me also saw it and knew it was real and very strange.

By now, I'm into my 50s and the fibers are everywhere, not just on me but everywhere around me, stuck to the headliner of my car and all around the house covering everything. When I wasn't struggling to keep my job I was struggling to clean everything I lived with. Sweat would pour out of me, as I sat doing nothing. I was in and out of Emergency

Rooms, suffering from toxic shock or dehydration. I carried an Epinephrine pen as an accessory. Morgellons would ravage my feet and legs 24/7 with crawling and biting. "Sounds like restless leg syndrome" the doctors would say. Right. Nights were spent scratching and getting in and out of the shower. My back felt like it was alive, living a separate life than my own. I realized that if I didn't find help I would soon end my life and move on.

So with a bit of help here and there I arrived at the end of my 57th year. Then something happened that turned my life around. The phone rang and a good friend screamed excitedly telling me to turn on the TV news channel. When I did I was hit like a bolt of lightening. There on the TV were pictures of my fibers and someone somewhere was treating it like a disease of the body! WOW! I thought at first this was a trick but soon found it to be the path to the next 8 years of a treatment.

Of course, the few medical professionals who were offering treatment knew very little about the *disease but at least they believed in it and were committed to helping. I was warned that since no hospitals accepted this as a "real" disease, treatment would take place at home and might make me feel better but could make me feel worse at first. Even if the treatment would make me worsen to the point of dying, it still sounded great, as long as I got a chance to call it by it's name and kick it's a**!*

So that's what I have been doing for about 8 years now and starting to see more improvements with each passing day. I had to retire from my job – yes, with all this going on I still managed to work nearly 35 years at the same place. Medical bills have eaten up my savings over the years but I do ok. The VA [veteran's administration] recently admitted me for care and medications so I am thankful for them.

Whatever causes Morgellons disease takes its time and doesn't rush to destroy the host. It sure brings about destructive behavior by those of us suffering with the disease since we are pre-judged by the medical community who seem satisfied with overlooking the physical illness and sending victims off to be placed on mental health watches. It's all very nerve-wracking to the newly infected, the freshly unclean, the shunned ones. Shunned people commit suicide rather than face another day of hearing "Now take it easy, you know the doctor said it's all in your mind".

Some people choose suicide, but not me. I am a fighter. The only fear I ever had was that when death came I would still not know this disease by name. One thing about antimicrobial drugs is that, given the right combination, you can actually get better. Eight years now and every day things change and when things turn bad it isn't long before there comes an overall improvement in my condition. I hear that treatment may last for at least as long as you've had symptoms. I seriously doubt that I'll live to be 130, so treatment for me is going to be for life.

Over the years I have lost numerous friends to all kinds of ways to die but the 5 that stick with me are the deaths of guys I grew up with living in northeast Los Angeles. Each and every one of the 5 had "undiagnosed bacterial infections" listed on the autopsy reports and nobody seemed surprised or even cared. Where are the medical people that look into this type of reporting or does it just get listed and forgotten? I don't see the CDC [Center for Disease Control] rushing out to check dead people who have "Undiagnosed bacterial infections". WHY NOT? Undiagnosed means that while alive these guys were infected and their doctor missed it. Boy, I can't wait to read my autopsy report. I wonder what percentage of the population has to die and have "undiagnosed" and "contributing" listed before someone at the CDC sits up and listens. I guess we'll have to wait and see.

Each day brings on new changes and new problems and nobody knows how this will end for me. I know that it took over 50 years for me to get the chance to fight this disease and for that I am thankful. Morgellons disease is still very much a mystery but it can only continue to hide if we continue to ignore those who suffer from its unforgiving rampage and the toll it takes on the victims it chooses to invade. I refused to be ignored or convinced that I was a mental case. I thank my Dad for that resolve and ask each of you to please not victimize the next person who tells you there are "strings" coming out of their fingers. Don't do what has been done before. Make the changes to change lives!

It's important that you understand that all of what I am saying here is personal, my opinions, my views and all true to me, a half-century in the making. The people who know me have always said: "if you don't want to hear the truth don't ask Bill". A very good friend of mine when asked why she always advises others to "ask Bill" replied, "Because when nothing seems right, crazy makes sense".

About 5 years into treatment with a specialist I dropped by my primary care doctor's office for a visit. The look on his face, the way he went speechless made all the nurses laugh. He said, "You've done it!" "It" being that I had proven to him that I wasn't nuts. But again that's just between him and me. It has not changed anything for the next person who suffers with Morgellons disease.

I can't tell you how many times I have been asked about what it has been like to live like this and survive in a world that seems to be against me. You come to accept the ignorance that surrounds you even when it costs you family and friends. It's part of the cost of being first on your block with an unknown disease.

About 2 years after I started treatment I entered my doctor's waiting room and it was full of sad, sick suffering people. After about 10 minutes a young girl was asked what she wanted out of treatment. She pointed at me and said, "I want to smile like he does". She had come from Australia to the U.S. looking for help. That was a while ago and I hope she got that smile she wanted. This is what Morgellons is and what it does and it happens every day somewhere and maybe even to somebody you love. We need to change the way we all look at the ways people suffer. We need to change ourselves to help others change as well.

From the writings of Bill Pitt

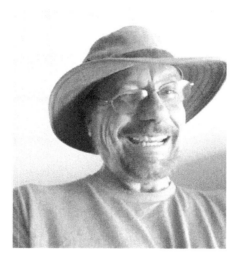

William Bruce Pitt

May 13, 1948 – January 29, 2015

RIP, Bill

Reading Bill Pitt's story, and the story of Cindy Casey in the first chapter, gives the reader a feel for the horror and isolation of Morgellons disease and introduces some of the disease's primary symptoms. Unfortunately, there are many more agonizing symptoms that MD patients share, one of them being insatiable and untamable itching all over the body. The next chapter discusses the phenomenon of itching, not only as a symptom, but also as a potential diagnostic sign of numerous diseases.

ITCHING: BOTH SIGN AND SYMPTOM

Fundamental to Morgellons disease is an intense urge to scratch, also known as itching or pruritis. Itching can either be the cause of a skin ailment (through scratching) or a result of it. Intense scratching can cause reddened or excoriated skin confounding the issue of cause versus effect. Many heath care providers persist in believing that the typical Morgellons lesions are a direct *result* of scratching even though patients continually report that the lesions appear independently. A basic review of pruritis as sign or symptom demonstrates its many causes.

Pathophysiology of Itching

Itching, like other skin sensations, is a self-protective mechanism. The itch sensation serves to warn the body of harmful external threats such as plants, insects, and parasites. The origins of itching can be dermal (irritation to the skin), neuropathic (due to damage to sensory nerves), neurogenic (originating in the central nervous system without evidence of nerve damage), psychogenic, or mixed. Itching can be elicited by external mechanical factors (e.g., insect bites, sunburn) or by internal, chemical mediators including histamine, neuropeptides, prostaglandins, tryptase, bradykinin, serotonin, acetylcholine, Substance P, Prostaglandin E, leukotrienes, or cytokines. Regardless of its cause, itching can be exacerbated by hot weather, psychological stress, skin inflammation, and skin vasodilation.

Itching and pain share a common neural pathway. Inflammatory mediators such as bradykinin have been shown to sensitize nociceptors (sensory nerve cells that transmit messages of discomfort to the spinal cord) for both itch and pain. The sensations of itching and pain interact antagonistically; the induction of pain (e.g., intense scratching, heat, or cold) inhibits itching through central mechanisms, whereas the reduction of pain (with centrally-acting opioid pain medications) enhances the itch sensation by disinhibition.

Itching as an Indicator of Systemic Disease

In the absence of a rash, itching can be an early indication of underlying systemic disease. Studies have shown that as many as 36% of pruritic patients have underlying systemic diseases and that itching is often the first symptom of the disease. Before initiating an investigation into the dermatologic, neurologic, or psychosomatic origins of a pruritic condition, the following systemic diseases should be considered: gall bladder disease, hepatitis, systemic lupus erythematosus, uremia, lymphoma, hypothyroidism, hepatitis C, human immunodeficiency virus, neoplasms, chronic lymphocytic leukemia, diabetes, hepatitis B, and iron deficiency anemia.

It is incumbent upon primary care providers, psychiatrists, and dermatologists to investigate the possibility of systemic diseases when patients complain of severe itching. Itching should never be considered psychopathic until systemic diseases have been ruled out. Unfortunately, Morgellons patients suffer many other symptoms besides intense itching. These will be reviewed in detail in the chapter that follows.

THE SYMPTOMS

The symptoms of Morgellons disease are unusual and unlikely-sounding and it is not surprising that anyone hearing about them for the first time would be doubtful and incredulous. I know that I was. The thing that made me a believer many years ago was the consistency of patients' descriptions of the exact same bizarre symptoms. When I first began seeing MD patients in my office there had been no media coverage of the disease and it was not being discussed on the Internet. It was implausible that this diverse group of patients was collaborating about what they were going to tell me! When I started to hear identical symptoms from dozens of people from all walks of life I began to pay attention and take a closer look at what was going on.

The following list of symptoms is based on data that I have collected over the years from hundreds of patients. There are actually more symptoms than are listed here but these are the ones that are most frequently reported. All patients have filaments but not all have every one of the following symptoms. In regard to the photographs, I know there will be disbelievers who think that the photographs have been altered or that the items that have already come out of the skin are actually debris found in the environment. However, I have seen all of these things in my office and know that the photographs you will see and the symptoms I am about to describe are very real.

1. Intense itching (this symptom has been reviewed in the previous chapter).
2. Disfiguring, spontaneously appearing, slow-healing lesions. In a small percentage, these lesions turn into large, deep wounds that will not heal.
3. Tough, difficult-to-remove scabs with keratin projections on the under side.
4. Blue, white, red, and black hair-like filaments extruding through the skin or seen just under

the epidermis using magnification. Some filaments are flattened and ribbon-like.

5. Thicker, translucent filaments that are visible without magnification and are very resistant to extraction.

6. Filaments that look like "feathers" because of the many fine projections from either side of the filament.

7. "Shards" of keratin that project down into the dermis causing pain until they are removed.

8. Black specks, "fuzz balls" and seed-like objects on clothing, skin and bed linens.

9. Hyper-pigmented, hypertrophic scars when the lesions first heal. These scars eventually become hypo-pigmented.

10. A waxy film on the skin all over the body as well as gobs of "gelatinous" material.

11. Occasional black tar-like exudate from the pores.

12. Metallic "glitter" on the face and other parts of the body.

13. Crystal-like exudates from skin.

14. A change in the texture or color of the hair.

15. Hair loss (to the point of total baldness in some).

16. An awareness of tiny flying insects around the body.

17. Blackening and crumbling of the teeth.

18. Fine markings on the skin that appear spontaneously but look like cat scratches or paper cuts.

19. Slightly raised, linear "tracks" on the skin.

20. What look like small "cocoons" coming from the scalp.

21. A soft, mushy "mound" on the crown of the head.

22. Susceptibility to static shocks and inability to wear watches or sit in front of a computer.

23. Systemic symptoms including profound fatigue, anxiety, insomnia, joint and muscle pain, headaches, loss of balance, dizziness and cognitive disturbances such as loss of short-term memory, and inability to concentrate or comprehend.

24. The constant and unnerving aggravation of feeling as though there are bugs or worms

crawling through one's body, biting, stinging, and causing unbearable discomfort.

As if the symptoms of the disease were not challenging enough, patients are forced to endure ridicule and abandonment by family, friends, and health care providers. Typically patients have futilely consulted as many as 20 to 30 different clinicians. With no hope in sight, it is no wonder that most Morgellons patients have depression, anxiety and/or suicidal thoughts and many have ended their lives. A discussion of what is currently known about the symptoms follows.

The lesions

The unusual thing about the lesions of MD is that they appear spontaneously although they look as though aggressive scratching may have caused them. Some patients do not have the lesions but the majority do and some have very few while others are literally covered by them. The lesions are very slow to heal and are therefore

71

unlike similar-looking lesions caused by other conditions. Another interesting aspect of these lesions is that they do not tend to develop secondary infections with *Staphylococcus aureus* or *Streptococcus pyogenes,* as would be expected if the lesions were caused by scratching.

Some patients report that a certain part of their body is particularly affected and covered with lesions. I have seen a predominance of lesions on the face, arms, hands, back and/or legs of the MD patients I have examined. For many patients the heavily affected area is the scalp. Patients have been known to shave their heads in an effort to keep hairs from becoming matted in the seepage from these open sores. Having a shaved head also facilitates application of topical medications or soothing creams to the lesions.

Patients have reported that when they apply a bandage to a lesion or even to a simple cut on the skin, the bandage becomes "shredded" by filaments. Total occlusion of the lesions seems to help them heal, at first, but when the occlusive dressing is removed the lesion and filaments reappear with a vengeance. At least 4 different types of pathogenic bacteria have been found in the lesions. This will be discussed in a later chapter when current research is reviewed.

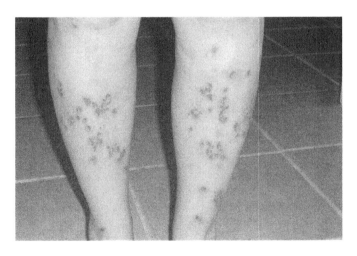

Image 1: Patients often present to the office looking like this. Color versions of all photographs in this book are available on www. gingersavely.com/morgellons-book.

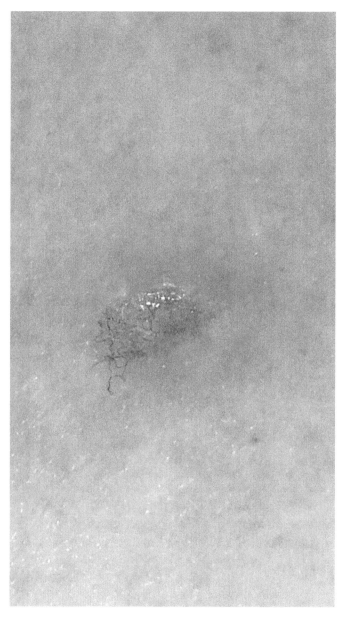

Iamge 2: Lesion with black filaments.

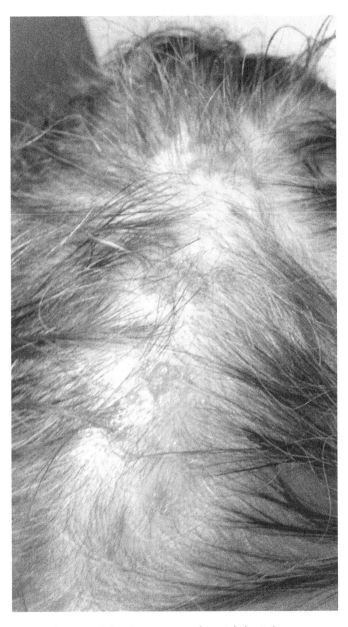

Image 3: Lesions on scalp with hair loss.

The Scabs

The tough scabs or calluses that form over many of the lesions not only contain masses of intertwined filaments of various colors but, most peculiarly, thick, firm, gelatinous projections on the inner side of the scabs as shown in the photos that follow. Using *Gomori Trichrome* stain, Middelveen and colleagues found these "plugs" (as patients refer to them) to consist primarily of keratin and to gradually harden in consistency over time. Significant pain relief occurs when patients are able to remove the scabs containing these projections. For this reason, patients are often seen picking, which is perceived as more evidence that the disease is psychopathic when relief of excruciating pain is the actual objective.

Of the following photographs, the first 3 show thin scabs containing intertwined filaments and the next 5 show tougher scabs with keratin projections or casts on the underside. Look carefully at these keratin projections that are found under the scabs of MD patients. I can think of no other human disease where something like this is seen and it would certainly not be expected in someone with a purely psychiatric disorder!

The photograph below, *Image 4,* when visualized in color, shows bright blue fibers intertwined within a patient's scab. See this photograph in color on www.gingersavely.com/morgellons-book.

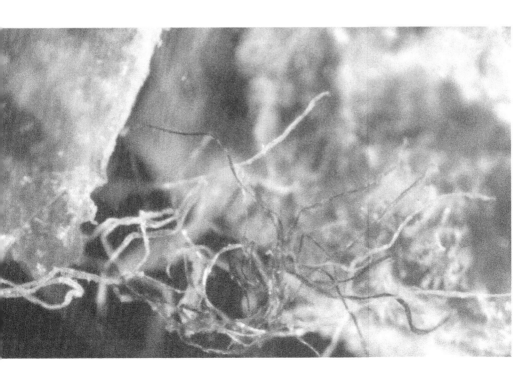

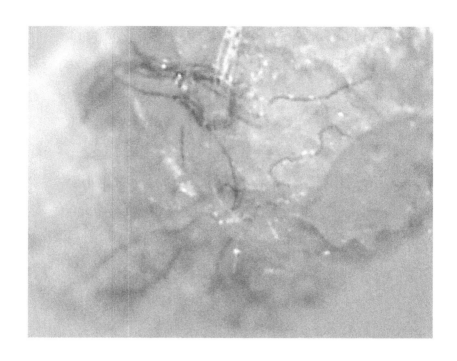

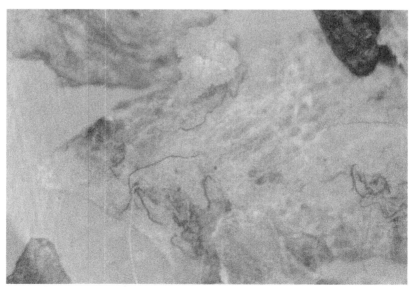

Images 5 and 6

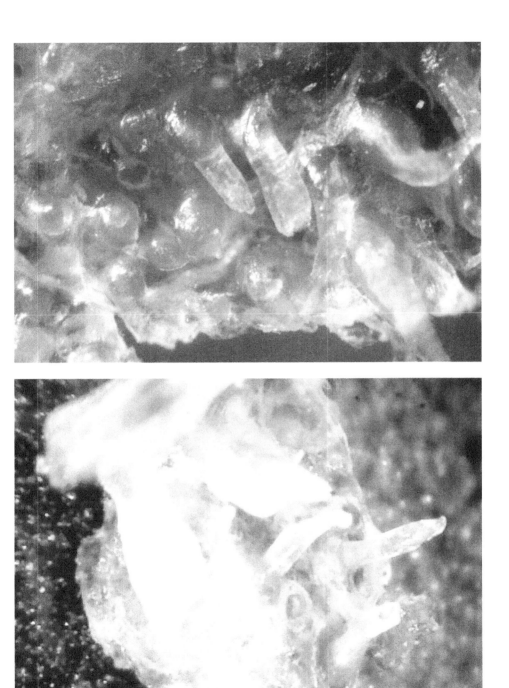

Images 7 and 8: Follicular casts seen at 100x magnification on the underside of removed calluses from MD patients.

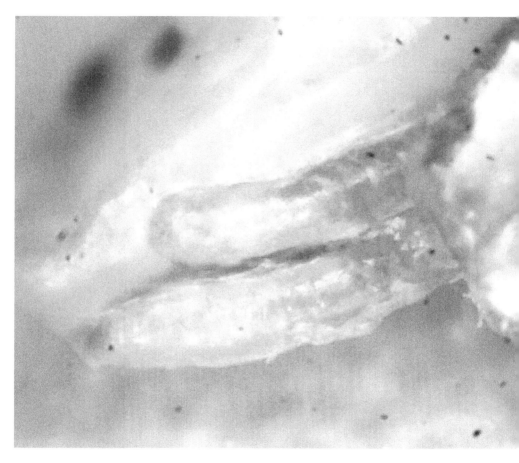

Images 9 and 10: Although these scabs showing keratin "plugs" were removed from one of my patients, they look very much like those seen in cows with Bovine Digital Dermatitis.

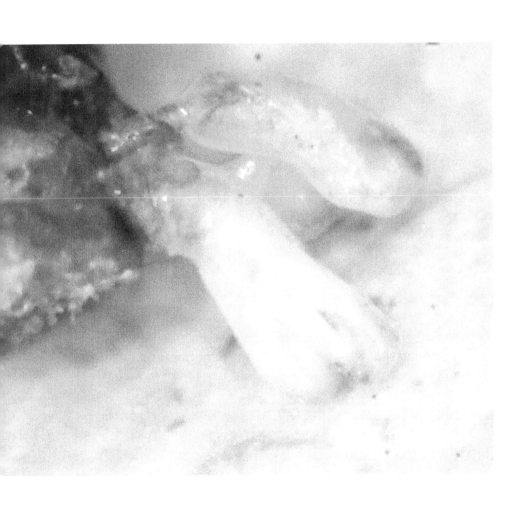

81

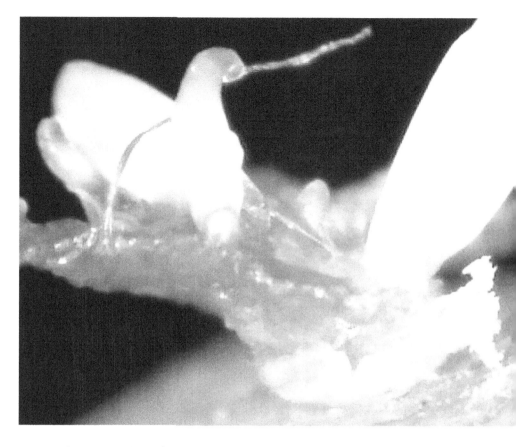

Image 11: A scab with keratin projections underneath as well as a filament that was growing down into the dermis.

Large, deep, non-healing lesions

A picture is worth a thousand words when it comes to this symptom. Photographs on the following pages are not for the faint of heart. Luckily, few MD patients have lesions this deep and large, although most patients have at least one smaller version of a deep lesion, which usually starts out as a circular "hole". I have primarily seen these types of lesions on the face but they can be on other parts of the body as well. Not surprisingly, facial lesions this dramatic are quite an embarrassment to the patient.

These deep wounds often appear to go down to the bone and they do not heal for many years. Wound care experts are baffled because every kind of wound healing method imaginable does not work. Biopsies reveal "non-identifiable fibers" and patients are accused of inserting these into their wounds. Interestingly, I have heard of several instances of these large wounds finally starting to heal once a biopsy is performed on them. I can only guess that the biopsy, being a new injury to the skin, stimulates the immune system to begin the healing process. There is no doubt that these wounds are like nothing ever seen before and are just one more peculiar aspect of this curious disease.

The following 5 photos are of an ill-fated male patient who suffered a series of these deep lesions. Unfortunately, this man's profession requires him to meet the public daily, making his appearance a constant source of embarrassment. The first photograph shows a hole on the left side of his face, the first of many deep lesions that appeared later in the same area. The next 3 photographs show the progression as the lesions take over the left side of his face. The fifth photograph shows what the area looked like after all the deep lesions he had suffered there had temporarily healed.

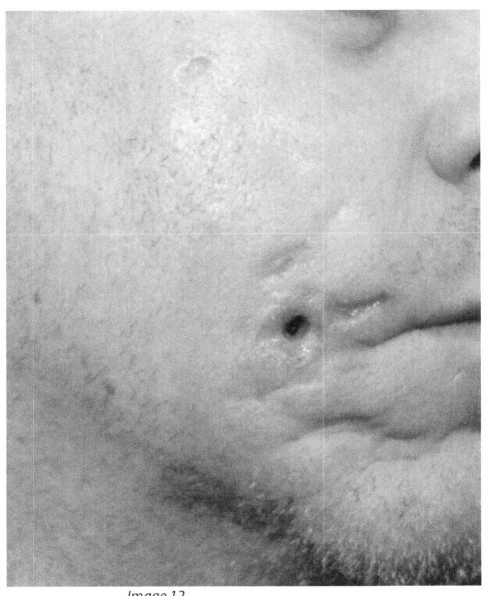

Image 12

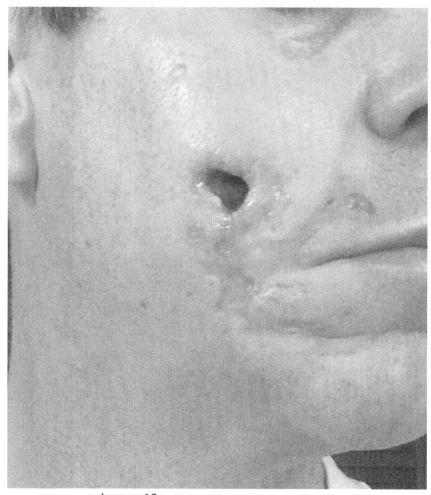

Image 13

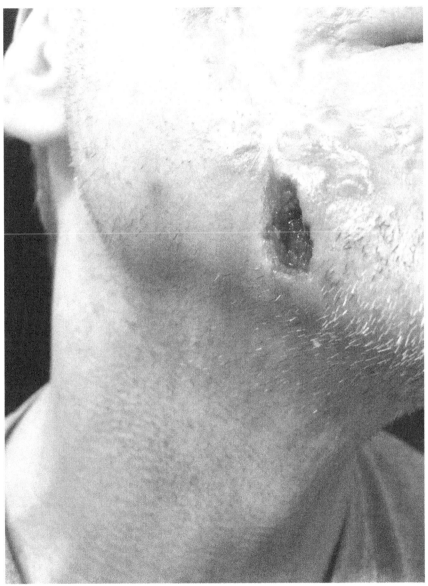

Image 14

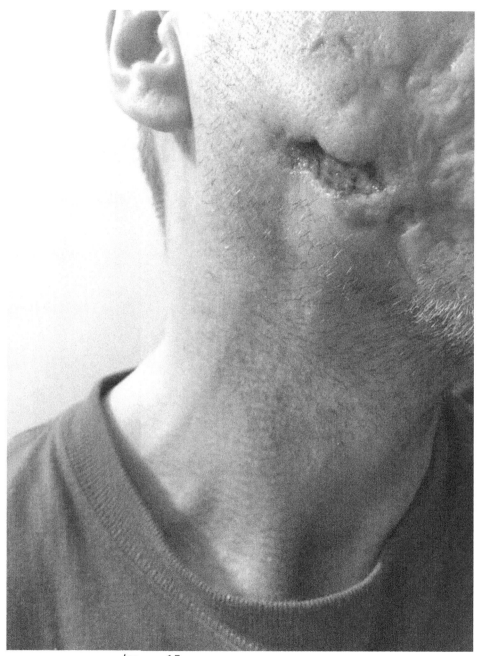

Image 15

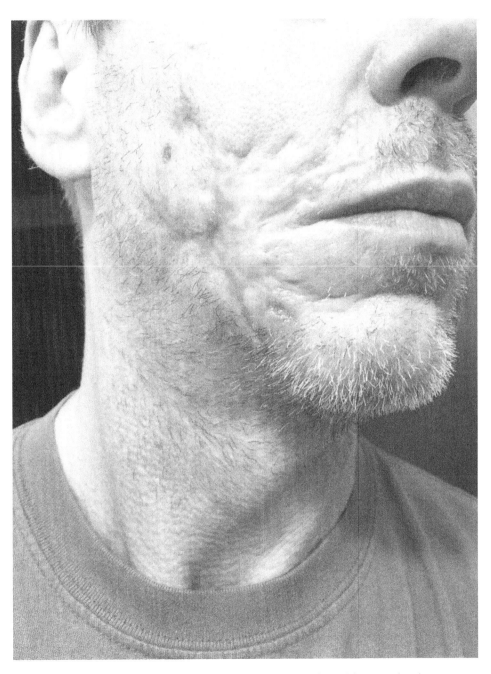

Image 16: Same patient after his numerous facial lesions had temporarily healed. Later his face opened up again in several new places.

Below is one of these deep lesions on the testicle of one of my patients (*Image 17*). If these wounds are self-inflicted (as many clinicians say they are) can you imagine that any man would want to do this to his testicle? Filaments and thick shards of keratin work their way through this patient's wound causing him extreme pain. He spends hundreds of dollars per month on

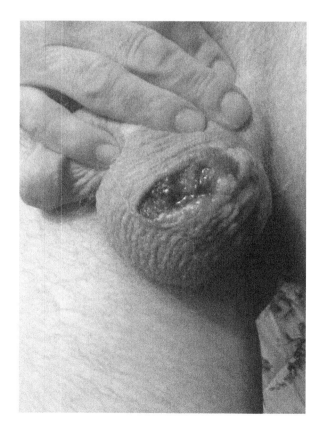

bandaging supplies because there is a constant sticky discharge from the lesion. This man had seen many specialists before he saw me and none of them were able to diagnose his problem or help him in any way. Most were downright insulting to him.

The filaments

Originally thought of as "textile contaminants" the filaments are now known to be composed of the body's own proteins, collagen and keratin, resulting from proliferation and activation of fibroblasts and keratinocytes in the epidermis and stemming directly from these cells. Collagen is the most abundant protein in the human body and is what holds the body together. Keratin is a key component of nails, hair and the outer layer of skin.

A problem for researchers is that textile fibers tend to attach themselves to the lesions and to the Morgellons filaments, adding confusion to the overall picture. Textile fibers actually do look like MD filaments under microscopy. It is only with the use of *Gomori Trichrome* and other specific stains that filaments can be clearly differentiated from textile fibers.

Filaments come out of MD patients' bodies in every way imaginable. They are in the mouth, gums, tongue and inner side of the cheeks. They come out of the eyes, ears and nose. Filaments are in urine and in seminal and vaginal secretions. They frequently grow out from under fingernails and toenails. Since a gastroenterologist told me that he has seen the filaments in the colons of 2 MD patients, there is every reason to believe they are present throughout the body. Interestingly, whenever an MD patient sustains an injury to intact skin such as an abrasion or even a paper cut, before long the injury becomes a new site of filament proliferation.

Researchers have seen retained cell nuclei at the base of filaments where they stem from the cell. Like human hair, on cross section MD filaments have a cortex and a hollow medulla. Using electron microscopy, the blue Morgellons filaments are shown to have scales much like a normal human hair. In contrast, some MD filaments have a smooth outer surface.

The filaments are thick and tough, fine and hair-like or flat and "ribbon-like". The thicker ones can be seen without magnification and I have always compared them to the look of nylon fishing line – translucent, tubular and very strong. These tougher filaments cannot be cut with scissors and are highly resistant to extraction. One of my West Texas patients said, "I wish I could market these filaments because I swear they would be strong enough to pull a tractor trailer".

The fine filaments can be black, white, blue or red and occasionally even orange, green, or purple. These filaments are nearly impossible to see without magnification. The fine filaments are strong as well: it is very difficult to obtain a punch biopsy from an MD patient since the intermeshed filaments will not break.

Patients have told me that of all the colored filaments, the red ones cause the most pain as they move through the skin. The red MD filaments are an unusual color of red and are actually more of a magenta/pink color. It is unknown how the magenta filaments get their color. The blue Morgellons filaments have been shown to contain granules of melanin, which may be responsible for their coloration. (Melanin is the pigment that gives color to human eyes, hair and skin.) Research has shown that the colors of the filaments are actual pigments rather than dye. Since dye is the origin of color in textile contaminants, this is one more piece of evidence that the filaments are **not** textile, as has been continually suggested by those who do not believe in the disease.

Many patients think that the filaments are alive and are infective agents. This is not the case.

The filaments are inanimate objects and are not capable of transferring MD to others. They may be thought of as by-products of the disease process. It is my assumption that there may be an electrostatic charge, which makes the filaments appear to move after they are extracted. Patients often refer to the filaments as worms, an unfortunate mistake that leads to further doubt and mistrust by their medical providers.

When I have tried to extract filaments of all kinds, MD patients describe a pain that radiates over an extended part of their body. The description I frequently hear is that it feels as though there is a connected web of filaments, so that when one is pulled it affects a larger network. These filaments are clearly not being implanted by the patient, as has often been suggested. Once doctors see these filaments for themselves and try to cut or extract them, they will be convinced that they are dealing with something very strange indeed.

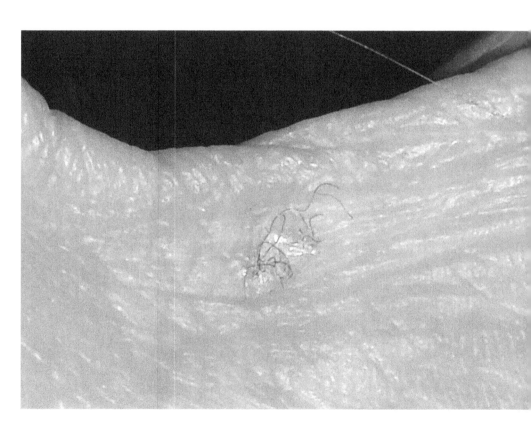

Image 18: Black and red filaments are seen in the web between a patient's thumb and forefinger. The color version of this photograph is on the book's front cover.

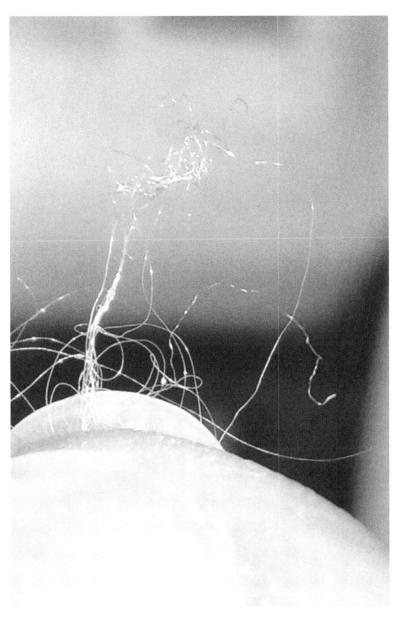

Image 19: Clear to white filaments are often seen growing from the underside of nails of MD patients.

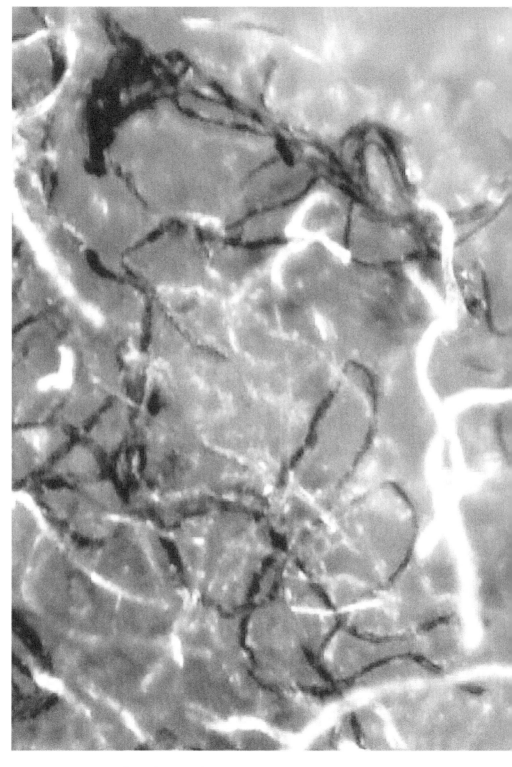

image 20: Black and white filaments as seen under the epidermis at 200x.

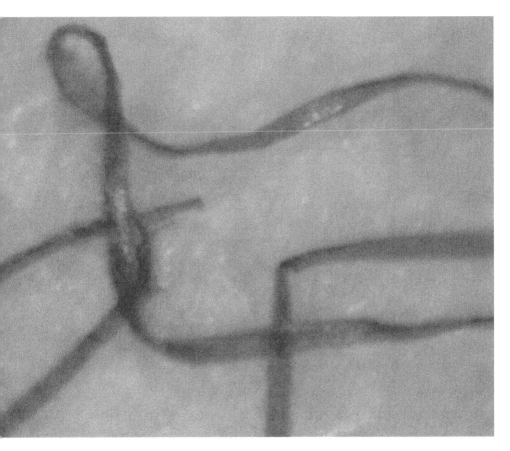

Image 21: A flat ribbon-like filament, this one from a vagina.

Feather-like filaments

It is not known why certain filaments have this appearance. Following this paragraph are a few photographs of this type of filament extruding from a patient's skin. When patients report that feathers are coming out of their body, health care providers understandably take this as evidence that they are mentally unstable. Rather than saying that feathers come out of their skin, patients need to be careful to say that they have filaments that vaguely resemble feathers. *(Image 22 below and 23 to the right).*

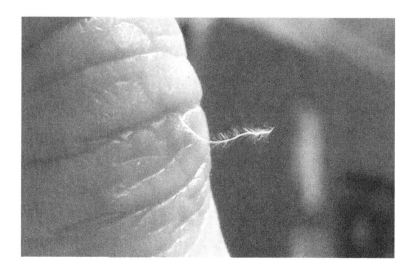

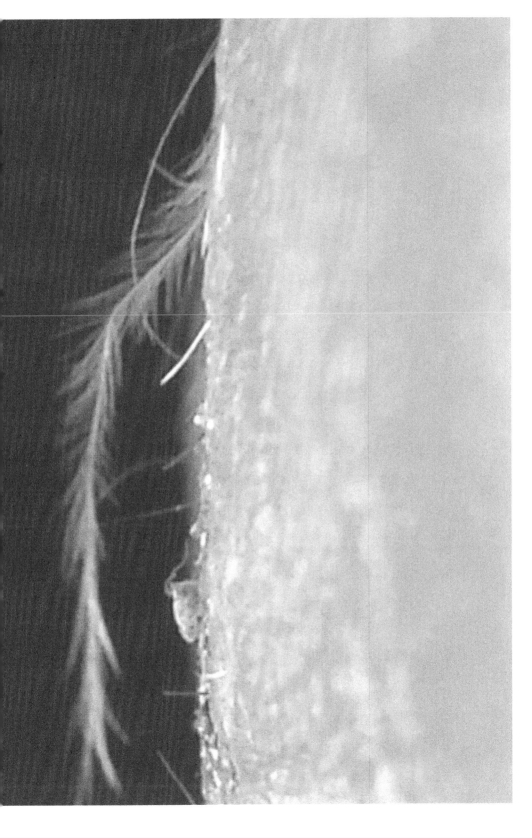

"Shards" of Keratin

Theses objects can vary in appearance but are a source of extreme pain for patients since they project down into the dermis. It is very difficult to remove them but patients are motivated to do so because once they are removed there is great relief of pain. I have seen hundreds of photographs of these objects through the years that patients have taken after they are finally successful in removing them. These shards are similar to filaments in the sense that they are made from the body's own proteins due to a proliferation of keratinocytes. Their size makes them more painful and difficult to remove than the filaments.

Images 24 and 25 are on the opposite page.

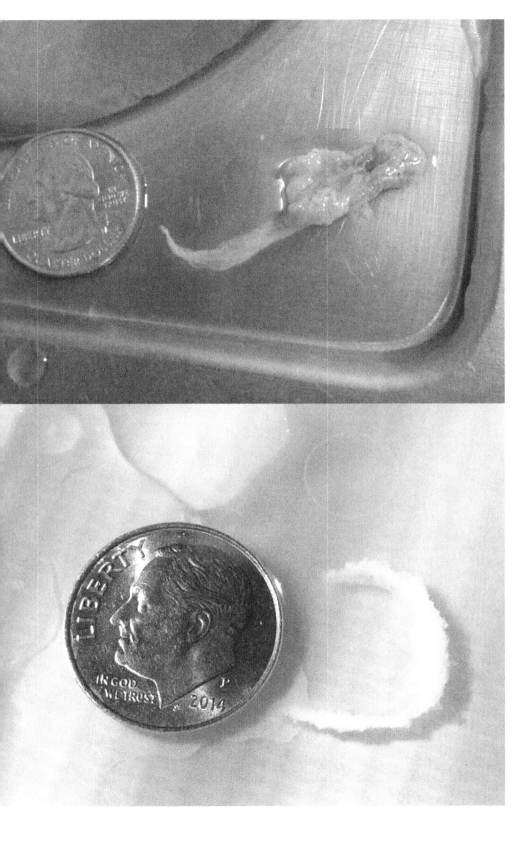

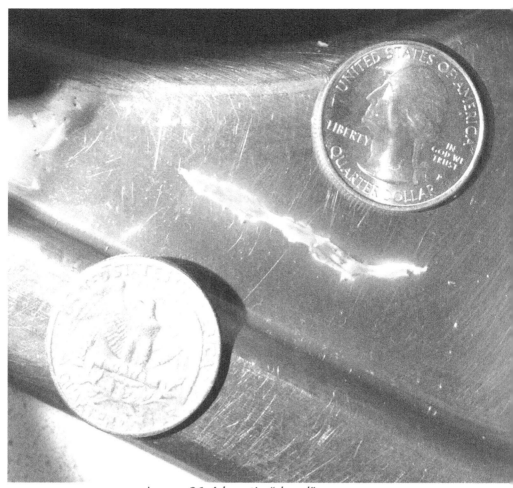

Image 26: A keratin "shard"

The black specks

Morgellons patients are sometimes accused of sprinkling ground black pepper or coffee grounds upon their skin when they complain of "black dots" on intact skin and in lesions. At the 2010 Morgellons disease conference Randy Wymore, M.D. presented slides demonstrating the difference between coffee grounds, pieces of ground black pepper and the black specks of Morgellons disease as seen by electron microscopy. The microscopy slides make it clear that the black specks are no more than black filaments coiled up into a tight ball, appearing upon magnification like a wound-up ball of string. On the other hand, Wymore's slides demonstrate that coffee and pepper sprinkles have sharp edges showing that they were cut by a grinder.

I have watched these black specks appear suddenly upon the skin of my MD patients. If the patient brushes the specks off of the skin they suddenly reappear. They may be coming through the pores of the skin but there is no proof of this. The black specks are definitely **not**, as some patients suspect, tiny insects that are responsible for their disease.

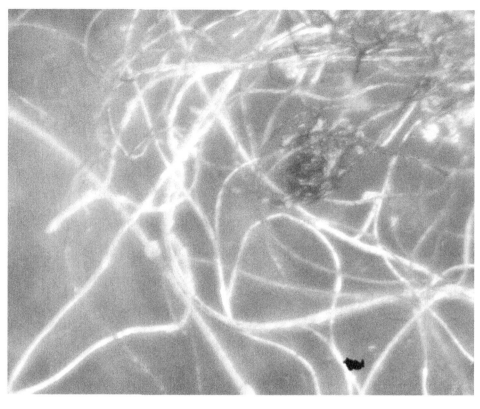

Image 27: A black speck amidst fibers in a skin sample from an MD patient. 70x magnification. Courtesy of M. Middelveen.

<u>"Fuzz balls"</u>

The fuzz balls, like the specks, are tangled masses of fine filaments but are looser with the appearance of tiny "dust bunnies". The following photo shows one of these fuzz balls at a magnification of 60x with the point of exit from the skin at 12 o'clock. (*Image 28*).

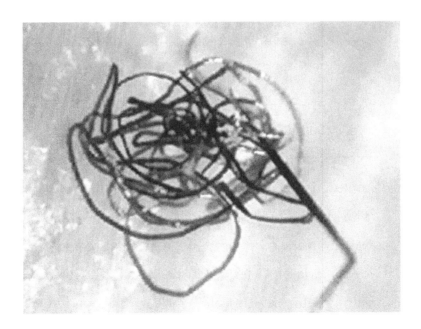

Gobs of gelatinous material

Morgellons patients report that there is gelatinous material coming out of their lesions and orifices. Clinicians and researchers have received samples from patients that become covered with what appears to be clear gelatin after remaining in a container. As mentioned in a previous paragraph, the scabs removed from MD patients' lesions have gelatinous projections on the underside of the scab, which become harder and more painful the longer the scab stays in place.

Some patients who believe they are infested with biting insects have erroneously confused the gelatinous plugs under the scabs with a type of larva or grub. Research shows that this is not the case; larvae are easy to dissect and identify. Hair follicles of MD patients are covered with gelatin, which can be clear, blue or red. Patients complain that their hair always looks dirty because of the exudate from their hair follicles.

The researchers Marianne Middelveen and Dr. Eva Sapi both surmise that the gelatinous material is likely alginate, an element of the biofilm produced by the bacteria found in the lesions of MD patients. I will discuss this further in the chapter on research.

The photograph below (*Image 29*) shows the slimy "goop" (as patients often refer to it) with embedded blue, red, white and clear fibers. As a

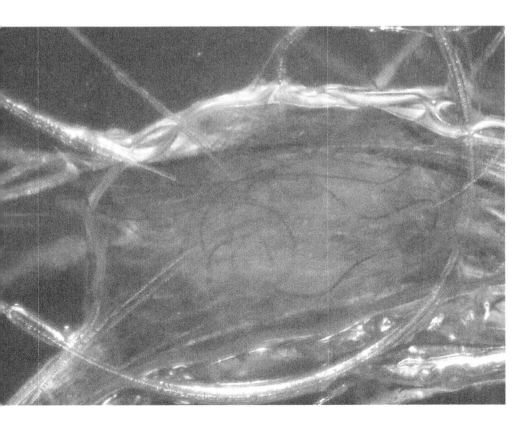

reminder, the color versions of these photographs may be seen on gingersavely.com/morgellons-book. Below, is a photograph of a single gelatinous plug from the underside of a small scab, immediately after having been removed by one of the CEHMDF nurses *(Image 30)*.

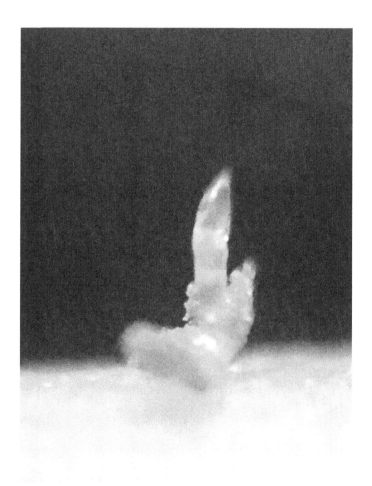

Film on the skin

We can only guess what causes the waxy film that patients report on their skin. Morgellons patients tell me that they feel like they should bathe four to five times a day because shortly after bathing they feel unclean again. I have heard this called "sticky sweats" and some even describe it as slimy. It has been postulated that the alginate that is a part of the gelatinous material may also be on the skin, causing this waxy feeling. We still do not have an explanation for this puzzling symptom.

I have wondered if there may be acidity to this waxy coating. Acidity on the skin would help explain the common complaint of MD patients regarding cotton clothing. Patients report that when they wear cotton socks or T-shirts they become covered with tiny holes after only one wearing. Many MD patients switch to wearing only clothes made with synthetic fabrics.

<u>Black tar-like liquid coming out of the skin</u>

About one-third of my MD patients report this symptom. Some say that this was one of their early symptoms that gradually disappeared over time. We do not know what this thick black liquid is or why it is present in some but not all of the MD patients.

One day as I was speaking with one of my MD patients in the office I recall seeing a bead of black liquid suddenly came out of one of the pores on her face. An MD patient once told me that when she went to the hospital to have a laceration sutured the doctor was horrified to see black fluid coming out of the lesion and stopped mid- procedure, refusing to continue. I have had a few patients show me that their brand new white socks were black after one wearing due to their feet being wet with "black sweat". Other MD patients have said that if they scratch their skin after they have been perspiring, they notice black fluid underneath their fingernails.

Image 31: The photo below shows this black liquid.

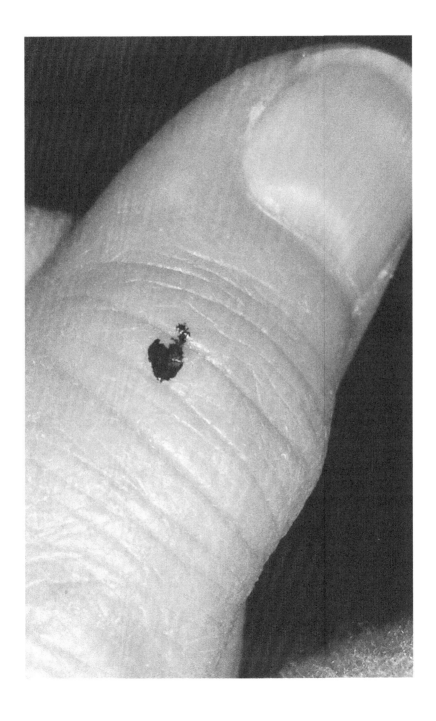

Glitter and Crystal-Like Exudates

This is one of the most puzzling and difficult-to-understand symptoms that MD patients report. I have seen the fine glitter myself on the skin of my patients, usually visible only under certain light. I think that the larger clumps

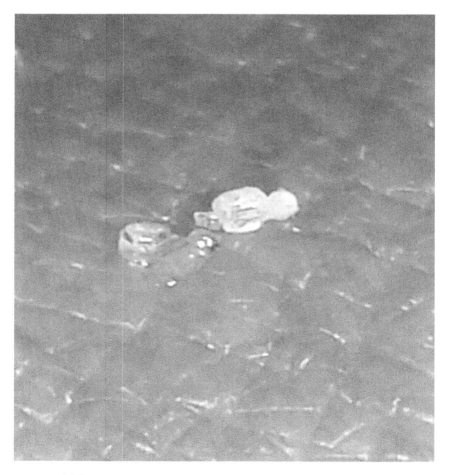

that resemble clear or opaque crystal are somehow related. Sometimes the little "crystals" are hard *(Image 32 on opposite page)*, other times they are so delicate and fragile that they disintegrate into dust. Patients have placed these crystals in bottles to send to researchers but the bottles arrive empty; the samples appearing to have vaporized. The researcher Marianne Middelveen plans to do x-ray crystallography of these exudates.

Change in the texture of the hair

At the 3rd annual Morgellons disease conference in 2010, Dr. Randy Wymore showed an electron microscope image of several hairs from the scalp of an MD patient that clearly showed a filament coiling itself tightly around each individual hair. This probably accounts for the change in hair texture that patients often complain about, saying that their hair has become thicker and coarser. If black filaments are coating the hair this also explains why MD patients sometimes say that their white or gray hair has turned dark again. "My hair is not my own" is something that I frequently hear from MD patients. Patients make this statement in an attempt to describe what is happening to them but unfortunately, it leads doctors to think that they are mentally unstable.

When black filaments grow out of the scalp and replace hair that is white or light blonde it may appear as though the hair has been dyed black. The short, white hair of one of my elderly male MD patients turned black, leading his friends to tease him about having dyed it. My patient knew that the black "hairs" that his friends were seeing were actually black filaments growing out of his scalp.

A complaint that I hear from patients who have long hair is that it can be perfectly combed and an hour later, even if the patient has been sitting still the whole time, there will be a tangled, matted mess of fine hairs at the nape of the neck.

Facial hair undergoes a change as well. Both male and female patients describe a thick growth of "peach fuzz" on their cheeks, in other words blonde, downy hair that is sometimes growing towards the ears instead of straight down. I have seen this on men and it is an entirely different type of hair than their normal beard growth.

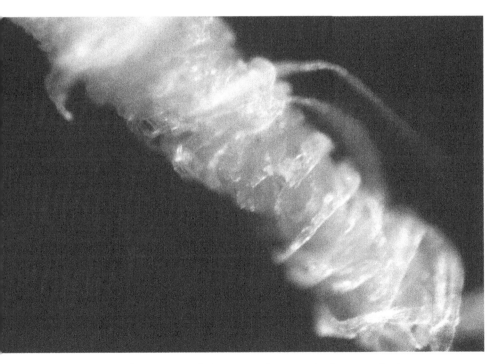

Image 33: Filaments tightly wound around a human hair at 200x.

Hair loss

Most MD patients report hair loss but only about 5% become totally bald. Some have a patch of baldness, usually on the crown of the head (a photo of this will soon follow). Hair may die and fall out because the filaments grow out of hair follicles and probably compete with hair for nutrients. Another possible reason is that the hair becomes brittle and unhealthy due to being encircled by filaments. My patients who have bought wigs to wear after suffering significant hair loss tell me that filaments growing into them cause a tangled mess, quickly ruining their wigs. I saw this for myself once when a patient removed her wig in my office.

Awareness of tiny insects flying around the body

About half of my MD patients share this complaint. Patients may indeed have an increase of tiny flying insects around them due to a different scent coming from their body but there is no way to know this for sure. Many of my Morgellons patients say that they have noticed a different and strange body odor since the initiation of their symptoms. Plus, there are the open, often oozing lesions that may somehow attract small insects. Unfortunately, some MD patients tell their doctors that these minuscule flying insects are the cause of their troubles, believing that the insects are laying eggs under their skin. However, none of the researchers believe that these insects are the *cause* of MD. It is very difficult to convince some MD patients that tiny flying insects are not the reason for their symptoms.

<u>Blackening and crumbling of the teeth</u>

Dentists have called me from all over the United States perplexed as to why patients with the symptoms of Morgellons disease have teeth that are black along the gum lines and falling apart. The teeth are not decaying; they are literally crumbling into pieces or becoming hollow on the inside so that they are nothing more than thin shells. We do not know why this is but I have had a hunch that whatever is causing MD may be leaching calcium from the body. I have also heard patients complain of tiny holes in their fingernails. It would be interesting to conduct research on this, looking at the dental records as well as the bone densities of MD patients.

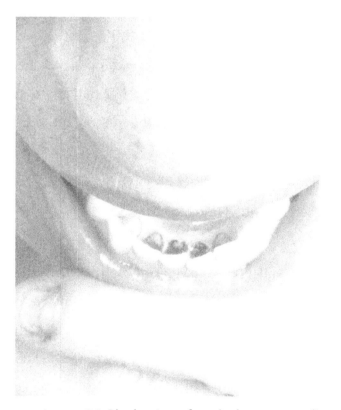

Image 34: Blackening of teeth close to gum line. Photo courtesy of Katie Yussuf.

"Scratch Marks" on the Skin

Below is a photograph of a woman's left breast showing an example of the mysterious "scratches" that spontaneously appear on MD patients' skin *(Image 35)*. Patients have actually watched as these markings occur right before their eyes. The explanation for these scratches is unknown but at times they do resemble the "striae" that are typical skin manifestations of Bartonellosis, as seen in the photograph that follows on the next page.

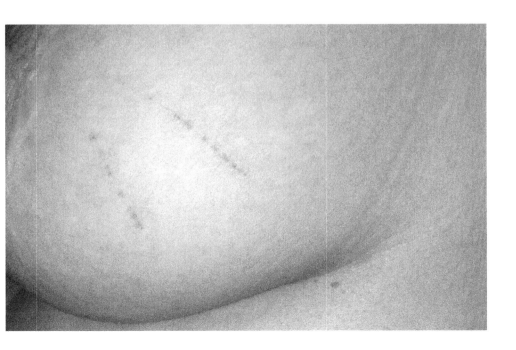

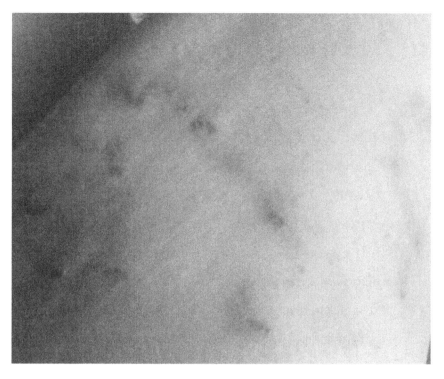

Image 36: Streaks on an MD patient's skin consistent with Bartonella striae.

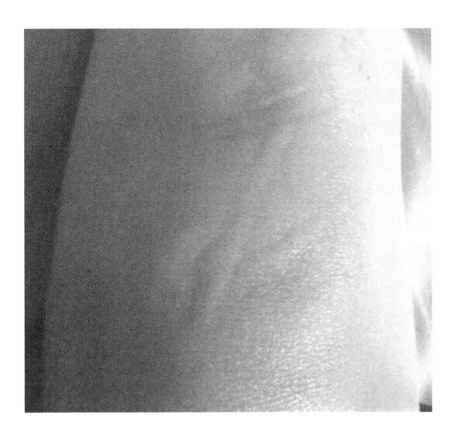

<u>Linear, raised "tunnels" or "burrows"</u>

These raised areas are the same color as
the surrounding skin and are not red, as would be
expected in someone with dermatographism (a
hypersensitivity reaction that occurs when
someone's skin is scratched and a red welt is left
exactly where the scratch mark was made). There

are no theories as to what causes this type of marking. The photograph below *(Image 38)* and the photograph on the previous page *(Image 37)* demonstrate this finding.

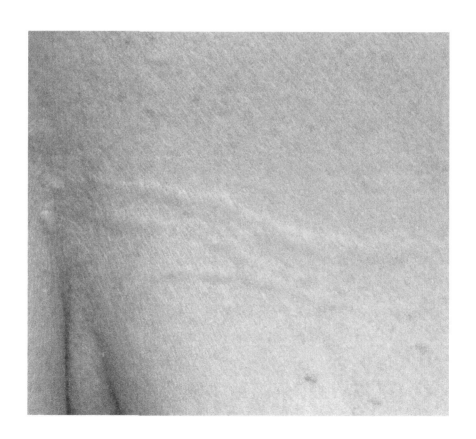

"Cocoons"

Morgellons patients shed material from their scalps that they believe to be "cocoons". Researchers have shown these to be follicular sheaths in which the filaments are forming. Often the filaments are tightly wound around the follicular sheath and can have the appearance of a small, white cocoon. It is important that patients not refer to these objects as cocoons, even if there is a strong resemblance, because this terminology can prejudice health care providers against them. A photograph follows *(Image 39)*.

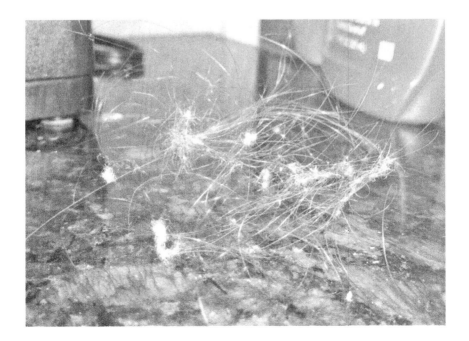

<u>Soft Mound on the Crown of the Head</u>

MD patients often complain of a soft mound on the crown of their head that feels "mushy" to the touch. This mound is a particularly intense area of all of the patient's unpleasant sensations. The soft, mushy feeling of this mound is believed to be due to the gelatinous material present in the base of the hair follicles. Below is a photo of one of my patients who shaved his head allowing this mound to be clearly seen. If a patient experiences partial balding it is almost always in this circular area at the crown of the head.

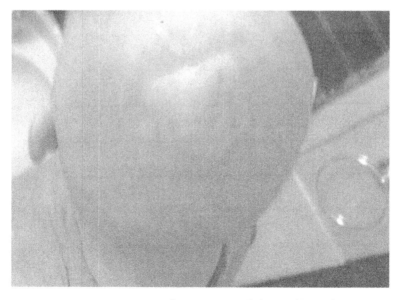

Image 40: Mound on crown of shaved head.

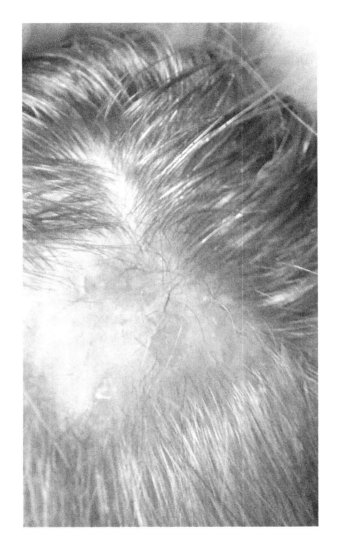

Image 41: Mound with lesions, showing loss of hair in that region.

In the case of only one of my patients this mound "erupted" into a round lesion, with a diameter of about 4 inches, deep enough to expose the skull. For cosmetic reasons, the patient convinced a plastic surgeon to surgically close the wound by. A few days after surgery the sutures burst open at which time my patient was accused of pulling them out herself. This allegation both shocked and offended her since she wanted nothing more than to have the unsightly lesion closed and had paid quite a bit of money to see that it was.

Crawling sensations under the skin

The crawling, biting and stinging sensations that MD patients experience are more than likely a combination of two processes. First, as the filaments push through and finally exit the body there is considerable discomfort due to injury to the skin. Patients have told me "I feel like I'm being stuck with pins but from the inside out". Also, a large part of the discomfort may be neuropathies caused by inflammation of the peripheral sensory nerves. Damaged small nerve fibers can cause sensations that are perceived as biting, stinging and crawling.

Due to the inflammatory nature of Lyme disease, Lyme patients who do **not** have MD often have feelings of crawling, biting and stinging as well. But, in the case of Lyme disease, these sensations are solely neuropathic in nature and there are no lesions or filaments. That which MD patients experience is far worse, because they actually have clear evidence of filaments working their way through the skin.

Propensity to static shocks and inability to wear watches or sit in front of a computer

I have noted clinically that a significant number of MD patients have below-normal levels of antidiuretic hormone (ADH), the hormone that gives a message to the kidneys to reabsorb some of the fluid that passes through them. Patients with low ADH have a condition called *Diabetes*

Insipidus (DI), an unfortunate name since it has nothing to do with "sugar" diabetes which is *Diabetes mellitus*. About 1 in 25,000 people in the general population develop DI but I see it to some degree or another in about a fourth of my MD patients. People with DI feel thirsty all the time and urinate frequently. They cannot stay hydrated because they eliminate fluids as fast as they drink them. These patients have saltier skin, which predisposes them to increased static shocks, a symptom often reported by MD patients.

Saltiness of the skin would also help explain the electrostatic movement that patients report when their filaments appear to move on their own as they protrude from the epidermis. It may also explain patients' reported inability to wear watches (because they stop) or sit in front of a computer screen (because they feel increased movement in their bodies when they do). This is all conjecture on my part.

Systemic Symptoms

Almost all of the MD patients I have treated have had systemic symptoms along with their skin symptoms. These symptoms are essentially the symptoms of Lyme disease and tickborne co-infections. The malaise and fatigue are profound. It is difficult to sleep and patients wake up in the morning feeling like a truck hit them. There is mental confusion including attention deficit, processing problems, and poor short-term memory. A new onset of anxiety and panic attacks is typical. There is pain in the joints and/or in the muscles. Many patients have neuropathies – nerves that are painful, burn, tingle or feel icy cold.

The list of tickborne infection symptoms experienced by MD patients goes on and on and includes cardiac symptoms like chest pain, shortness of breath and palpitations; gastrointestinal symptoms like abdominal pain, nausea and diarrhea; urinary symptoms like frequent and painful urination; and neurological symptoms like muscle twitching, dizziness, loss of coordination, hypersensitivities and difficulty walking.

A comprehensive list of the symptoms of Lyme disease, available at www.lymedisease.org will leave the reader amazed to see dozens of symptoms affecting every body system. The fact that MD patients experience so many systemic symptoms that are typical of Lyme and other tickborne diseases strengthens the speculation that MD is a physiological rather than a psychosomatic illness and that it has some kind of connection with tickborne infections.

Summary

After hearing about the symptoms of Morgellons disease you are either eager to continue reading to find out more about this enigmatic disease or you have decided to put this book down, having reached the conclusion that the writer has lost her mind. I hope that your decision is not the latter, although I certainly wouldn't blame you if it were. Please have faith that what you are about to learn will be eye opening, even though at times disturbing and unbelievable. If it is difficult to read about the symptoms of MD and see photographs of its ravages, only try to imagine how dreadful it must be to be one of its victims, suffering not only the pain of the symptoms but the indignity of being labeled a drug abuser or a delusional psychotic. The next chapter will discuss these two diagnoses, the most common misdiagnoses conferred upon Morgellons patients: drug-induced formication and delusions of Parasitosis.

THE MOST COMMON MISDIAGNOSES

The conditions most often confused with Morgellons disease are drug-induced formication and delusions of parasitosis. Both of these diagnoses are frequently given to MD patients who present to hospital emergency departments in a state of panic, agitation, and extreme discomfort.

Drug-induced Formication

Drug-induced formication is a sensory hallucination initiated by psycho-stimulant drugs such as cocaine or amphetamines. Abusers of psychostimulant drugs often have a sensation of bugs crawling all over their bodies, referred to as "coke mites," "meth mites," or "amphetamites" depending upon the offending agent. Patients with this drug-induced disorder often create open lesions on accessible areas of their skin due to picking and scratching. Morgellons patients who present to hospital emergency departments covered with lesions and complaining of "bugs" biting them are usually accused of being drug addicts.

The majority of patients with Morgellons disease have no history of psycho-stimulant drug use and their skin lesions appear spontaneously. Most importantly, MD patients, as opposed to patients with drug-induced formication, have filaments that perforate their skin in locations throughout the body, including areas that a patient would not be able to reach with his own hands.

Delusions of Parasitosis (DOP)

In the late 19th and early 20th century medical literature, the condition that we now know as DOP was referred to as parasitophobia (fear of parasites). Karl-Axel Ekbom, MD, a Swedish neurologist, proposed a new way of thinking about the condition in his 1938 paper published in *Acta Psychiatrica et Neurologica Scandinavico.* Ekbom, whose legacy includes the naming of the condition "Restless Leg Syndrome", published a literature review and seven detailed case histories of Scandinavians diagnosed with parasitophobia. He pointed out that none of the patients whose cases he described suffered from sensory misperceptions, delusions of reference, grandiosity, substance abuse or symptoms of schizophrenia, as would have been expected had they truly been delusional.

Ekbom cautioned that a delusional diagnosis should never be given to a patient without first performing a thorough physical exam. He advised against the further use of the term parasitophobia pointing out that none of these patients had a **fear** of having bugs in their skin – they were **sure** that they had them. Since most of the patients in Ekbom's review of the parasitophobia literature ranged in age from 50 to 70, he proposed a new name for the condition - "Presenile Delusion of Infestation".

Apparently, the new name did not catch on. In fact, after the publication of his 1938 paper, the disease began to be known as Ekbom's Syndrome. It is unfortunate that his name became associated with a delusional condition since Ekbom specifically wrote that he did not believe these patients to be delusional (it is not clear why he used the word in his proposed new name). In fact, he surmised that these supposedly delusional patients had legitimate physical symptoms (probably paresthesias) that they perceived incorrectly. Ekbom stated his case that these patients are not delusional by making the following points:

1. "The symptoms are concrete, detailed and convincingly described." Furthermore, the symptoms do not fit neatly into any of the diagnostic criteria for psychiatric illnesses.
2. Each patient reports that symptoms are worse in a certain part of their body and they do not waver in this description.

3. Some patients do not blame their symptoms on insects or other pests.
4. Scratching does seem to temporarily alleviate the itch.
5. The sensations remain unchanged for long periods of time.
6. Most patients are able to distinguish between their complaints and their interpretations (can be convinced that the symptoms are not due to "bugs").
7. The symptoms can disappear with a change in environment.
8. A single hallucination not accompanied by other psychiatric symptoms is very rare.

It is interesting that of the seven cases Ekbom described, three reported a history of syphilis, a disease that was rare in Sweden. He did not know what to make of this finding although he did point it out in his paper. Ekbom made reference to a 1935 paper by J. Vie in which six of eight reported cases of this "delusional" infestation reported a history of syphilis. This association is fascinating considering that syphilis is caused by the spirochetal bacterium *Treponema pallidum*, the cork-screw-shaped first cousin of *Borrelia burgdorferi* that causes Lyme disease.

I was stricken by the fact that in all of the reported cases, despite detailed descriptions of physical exams, patients' skin was never examined with lighted magnification. Furthermore, the fact that Ekbom's patients did not complain of filaments suggests that they may not have had MD. As will be discussed in the next chapter, people who have neurological paresthesias (unusual sensations caused by damaged nerves), including biting, crawling and stinging sensations, do **not** have MD if they do not have filaments. In fact, I am often asked if I diagnose everyone with Morgellons disease who comes to me expecting that they have it. The answer is no, because some of these patients have paresthesias without filaments and therefore do not qualify for an MD diagnosis.

In the DOP literature, one learns that DOP patients often refuse to accept a psychiatric diagnosis for their skin symptoms, and continue to insist that they have a parasitic infestation. In medical school, physicians learn about the "matchbox sign" of DOP, so-called because patients used to bring samples of "hair," "lint," or "fuzz" to the physician in a matchbox in an attempt to provide evidence of the agent responsible for their torment. When two people describe symptoms of DOP, the condition is termed *folie à deux* (madness of two). *Folie à trois* (madness of three) and *folie à quatre* (madness of four) may also occur. Delusional parasitosis affecting all members of a family is considered *folie à famille* (madness of family). A new term, *cyberchondria* describes those who become so sympathetic to what they read about a disease on the Internet that they begin to have the symptoms themselves.

Morgellons disease differs from DOP in a number of ways. First, MD is seen in children and children are not known to develop delusional disorders. Second, DOP occurs in patients with normal physical functioning, whereas almost all Morgellons patients have significant impairment in physical functioning. Finally, the association with *Borrelia burgdorferi* and other bacteria suggests that Morgellons disease has a somatic rather than a psychiatric etiology.

Antipsychotic medications such as *pimozide* or *risperidone* are often prescribed for DOP patients but are rarely effective. It has been postulated by psychiatrists that the reason antipsychotics are not helpful is that patients are reluctant to take them as directed. Of course, the other obvious possibility is that they do not work because the patient is not psychotic!

The diagnosis of DOP is rare in the United States with a prevalence estimated at 2.37 to 17 per million per year. It affects both sexes equally beneath the age of 50 but over the age of 50 the male to female ration is 1:3. The most common age of onset ranges between 55 to 68 years. The average duration of DOP is 3 years with symptoms resolving spontaneously. In some cases, it may last for decades. There are no particular predilections for DOP and patients have no prior history of psychiatric problems. Many sufferers are high functioning, intelligent professionals including doctors, lawyers, and psychologists.

A review of the literature on DOP reveals a couple of other interesting findings about DOP: 1) onset is more likely in warm weather months, and 2) onset usually occurs after a severe psychological stress. So, in review, we are looking at a condition that has always been very rare but is now increasing in incidence, that is seasonal, that follows immune-suppressing stressful events, that happens to people with no psychiatric history, that resolves spontaneously in some of its victims, and that may occur in more than one family member at a time. This sounds more like an infection than a delusion, does it not? In fact, a recent explosion in the number of patients with the symptoms of Morgellons disease has given rise to a virtual epidemic of "Delusions of Parasitosis". The sudden prevalence of DOP raises suspicion that these unfortunate people may actually have had a real, unrecognized disease all along.

Relationship of Morgellons Disease to Psychopathology

The psychopathology observed in Morgellons patients appears to be attributable to the disease itself, with the disease ultimately affecting the ability of some patients to distinguish reality from delusion. This aspect of the disease might be compared to the clinical course of infection with *Treponema pallidum*, the spirochetal cause of syphilis, which in the early stages exhibits skin manifestations, and left untreated, can result in severe neuropsychiatric pathology. Unfortunately, when a patient presents with obvious psychopathology there is a tendency on the part of the clinician to assume that the psychopathology is the primary rather than secondary condition.

The syphilis model highlights a basic premise of psychosomatic dermatology: the diagnosis of a delusional disorder must be based on the presence of a primary psychiatric illness rather than the absence of known disease. At the 2016 Morgellons disease conference in Austin, Texas, Robert Bransfield, M.D., a psychiatrist who specializes in treating Lyme disease patients, gave a presentation in which he stressed that a psychiatric diagnosis should never be a diagnosis of exclusion. If a health care provider is unable to narrow down the cause of a patient's symptoms, an automatic referral to psychiatry is not appropriate.

The prevalence of delusional disorders in the United States is estimated in the *DSM-5* to be about 0.02% and the prevalence of mood disorders about 5% (American Psychiatric Association, 2013). Dr. Bransfield reviewed the backgrounds of 3000 self-reported cases of MD and found pre-existing delusional disorders and mood disturbances to be no more prevalent than would be expected in the general population. In the case of MD, it has been my conjecture, based on clinical observation, that the factor inducing the skin disease triggers secondary psychopathology that may be erroneously confused with a primary delusional disorder.

Thus, when psychopathology is observed in MD patients it is the result of the disease rather than the cause of it. I have noted that patients often develop OCD (Obsessive-Compulsive Disorder), becoming obsessed with their affliction and compulsive about removing their painful filaments. Patients become extremely anxious and a new onset of panic attacks is common. Many MD patients are diagnosed with ADD (Attention Deficit Disorder) because of the cognitive dysfunction that is a symptom of their illness. I roughly estimate that about a third of MD patients develop some degree of bipolar disorder, fluctuating between severe depression and hypomania. I do not have statistics on the development of psychopathology in MD patients but the CEHMDF and I have observed that a small percentage of patients ultimately become paranoid delusional. In these situations, a psychotropic medication can assist the patient in coping with the disabling anxiety stemming from the delusions. The psychotropic medication will not cure their disease but it will help the patient to more calmly approach what they need to do in order to heal.

Drug-abuse and DOP are not the only misdiagnoses conferred upon Morgellons patients even though they are the ones most frequently made in urgent care situations. The next chapter reviews the many different skin conditions that may be confused with Morgellons disease and the ways in which each of these skin diseases differs from this new filament disease.

DIFFERENTIAL DIAGNOSIS OF MORGELLONS DISEASE

When a patient presents to a health care provider with an array of symptoms, the first thing the practitioner does is to formulate a differential diagnosis. The "differential" (it is usually shortened this way) includes all of the conditions with similar symptoms that need to be ruled out in order to arrive at a correct diagnosis. For example, the differential for abdominal pain is extensive including, but not limited to, irritable bowel syndrome, gastroenteritis, appendicitis, gallstones, diverticulitis, mesenteric thrombosis, or cancer.

Morgellons disease is almost always misdiagnosed leading to prolonged suffering for the patient and a reduced chance of recovery. It is important to review the differential diagnosis for Morgellons disease because it is essential to understand the differences between MD and other similar skin diseases. Included in this differential diagnosis are psychosomatic, drug-induced, allergic, neurologic, metabolic, autoimmune, and primary or secondary infectious dermatological processes.

Systemic diseases, as discussed previously, should be ruled out before investigating the cause of any skin condition. The psychosomatic and drug-induced conditions in the differential were reviewed in the last chapter: drug-induced formication and delusions of parasitosis. The rest of the dermatological differential will be listed below, focusing specifically on skin conditions that are characterized by itching, multiple lesions, and pervasive discomfort.

Contact or Atopic Dermatoses

Xerosis

Also called asteatotic eczema, xerosis is the name for skin that itches due to dryness and flakiness. Xerosis occurs more often in older adults and during the winter months. Patterns of redness are observed in the areas that are most frequently scratched.

Allergic contact dermatitis

Contact dermatitis occurs when a patient comes in direct contact with a substance that is an allergen. Common culprits are cosmetics, laundry detergents, latex, nickel, and poison ivy or oak. Contact dermatitis rashes are confined to the exposed area and vary in severity according to the dose per unit area exposed.

Atopic dermatitis

Referred to as the "itch that rashes", atopic dermatitis is a skin manifestation of systemic allergy, usually occurring in those with a personal or family history of allergies or asthma. The presence of a profuse or highly localized area of dryness or redness, rather than intradermal filaments and discrete, randomly located lesions, differentiates Morgellons disease from rashes due to xerosis, allergic dermatitis, or atopic dermatitis.

Neurological Dermatosis

Cutaneous Sensory Disorder (Cutaneous dysesthesia). Patients with diabetes and certain neurotoxic infections may experience paresthesias, which include feelings of crawling, biting, stinging, and profuse itching. The condition is sometimes known as cutaneous sensory disorder. In contrast to Morgellons patients, these patients have no visible skin manifestations and no filaments or other unusual objects extruding from their skin. Even Lyme disease patients who do **not** have Morgellons disease often have paresthesias.

Hereditary or Disease-Associated Dermatoses

The **perforating dermatoses** are a group of skin diseases characterized by the elimination of elastic or collagen fibers from the upper dermis through the skin and include the following five diagnoses: Kyrle's disease, perforating folliculitis, reactive perforating collagenosis, elastosis perforans serpiginosa, and acquired perforating dermatosis. The perforating dermatoses are associated with hereditary diseases including Ehlers-Danlos syndrome, osteogenesis imperfecta, Down's syndrome, and Wilson's disease. They may also be seen in patients with brittle diabetes mellitus or dialysis-dependent renal failure.

The perforating dermatoses are distinct from Morgellons disease because the protruding filaments are made up of elastic or collagenous tissue that is easily identified by histopathology. In addition, Morgellons patients rarely have the unusual hereditary conditions or severe metabolic abnormalities associated with the perforating dermatoses. Conversely, systemic and neuropsychiatric symptoms have not associated with the perforating dermatoses, and they do not respond to antimicrobial therapy.

Skin Conditions with Infectious Causes

The differential diagnosis for Morgellons disease includes the following skin infections: Scabies; bed bugs; Tropical Dermatoses; Strongyloides; Cutaneous Leishmaniasis; Bacillary Angiomatosis; Endemic Treponematoses and Herpes Zoster. A review of these dermatoses follows.

Scabies

Scabies is a transmissible skin infection caused by infestation with the microscopic mite *Sarcoptes scabei* and characterized by extreme itching at night, superficial burrows, and a secondary hypersensitivity reaction. The infestation is found primarily in the webbing between the fingers and in the skin folds on the wrist, elbow, or knee. MD patients are often misdiagnosed with scabies at first but the lack of the typical scabies skin distribution or mite infestation, the absence of easy person-to-person transmission, and the presence of filaments distinguishes Morgellons disease from scabies.

Bed Bugs

Bed bugs (*Cimix Lectularius*) are parasitic insects of the Cimicid family that feed exclusively on blood. Many Morgellons patients are misdiagnosed with bed bugs or are convinced that that is what they have after researching on the Internet. It is easy to see how this mistake could be made since both are typified by very itchy lesions with the sensation of something crawling under the skin. I did once remove a bed bug from an MD patient's lesion but I am sure that it had adhered to the patient's sticky lesion when she had come in contact with it. People suffering from bed bugs do not have the filaments in their lesions that are characteristic of Morgellons disease.

Tropical Dermatoses

The tropical dermatoses are caused by parasitic infections, including filariasis, onchocerciasis, and cutaneous larva migrans. These dermatoses are prevalent in the tropics, and the skin lesions are associated with eosinophilia (elevation in a specific type of white blood cell), lymphatic obstruction (in filariasis), subcutaneous nodules (onchocerciasis) or serpiginous skin lesions (larva migrans). Diagnosis is made when the causative nematode is detected in skin biopsy samples. In contrast, eosinophilia is not reported in Morgellons patients, and nematodes have not been identified in skin biopsies of Morgellons patients. However, the tropical dermatoses may respond to treatment with anthelminthic medications (used to treat worms and nematodes) such as ivermectin and thiabendazole and anecdotally, antihelmintic therapy has been shown to be useful in treating Morgellons disease.

Strongyloides stercoralis

Many of the MD patients I have examined have been convinced that they are infested with *Strongyloides* parasites, commonly known as threadworms. It has been my experience, that when Morgellons patients are treated with ivermectin, the drug of choice for threadworms, many report a decrease in symptoms. However, Morgellons disease patients do not have stool cultures that are positive for ovum or parasites, and the filaments found in the skin of Morgellons patients are not worms, but rather inanimate objects.

Cutaneous Leishmaniasis (CT)

CT is a skin infection caused by one of about twenty different species of the leishmania protozoa and transmitted through the bite of a female sandfly. The disease may present viscerally, although the cutaneous (skin) form is more prevalent. CT occurs primarily in the Middle East,

Northern Africa, and in the Americas from Texas to Argentina. The presence of ulcerated lesions, which form atrophic scars, is one characteristic CT shares with Morgellons disease. However, CT is rare in the United States (in the absence of recent travel history to an endemic region), the lesions are not painful as they are in Morgellons disease (unless they become secondarily infected), and there are no filaments reported or visualized on exam.

Bacillary angiomatosis (BA)

Caused by a cutaneous or visceral infection with the bacteria *Bartonella henselae* or *Bartonella Quintana,* BA is characterized by red, sometimes ulcerated, papules or nodules all over the body. In my experience many MD patients do test positive for antibodies to one of the *Bartonellas,* however, BA usually responds dramatically to the antibiotics doxycycline or erythromycin whereas MD does not. The appearance of BA may be similar to that of Morgellons disease, however, a careful examination of BA lesions with magnification does <u>not</u> reveal the filaments characteristic of MD patients.

The Endemic Treponematoses

The endemic treponematoses are forms of non-venereal syphilis and include *yaws*, *bejel*, and *pinta*. They are caused by spirochetes of the genus *treponema* and they all manifest in multiple stages involving the skin. Although three different kinds of spirochetes have been found in the lesions of MD patients, *B.Burgdorferi*, *H.pylori and T. denticola*, the specific *treponema* spirochetes responsible for the endemic treponematoses have not been found in tissue biopsies of MD patients.

Herpes zoster

Commonly known as shingles, herpes zoster is a painful and pruritic cluster of vesicular (fluid-filled) lesions and is a reactivation of the varicella-zoster virus, which resides in the nerves long after the patient's first infection with the virus ("Chicken-pox"). Unlike Morgellons lesions, the lesions of shingles are vesicular and tend to erupt along neural dermatomes. Shingles usually resolve spontaneously but the disease course may be ameliorated by anti-viral medications. In contrast to MD, there are no filaments in zoster lesions.

Dermatoses Secondary to Skin Trauma

The diagnoses in the differential that are skin problems resulting from scratching or other trauma are folliculitis, prurigo nodularis, and impetigo. A discussion of each of these conditions follows.

Folliculitis

Folliculitis is a minor infection that starts in the hair follicles and often occurs in both men and women in body parts that have been shaved. Raised, inflamed, bumps may occur all over the affected area. Morgellons patients are often misdiagnosed with folliculitis because at first glance there is a similarity between the two conditions. However, Morgellons lesions occur sporadically all over the body, and not necessarily in shaved areas, and contain the characteristic filaments that are lacking in the lesions of folliculitis.

Prurigo Nodularis

The cause of prurigo nodularis is unknown and therefore it is unclear as to whether it is a skin infection in its own right or one that is the result of intense itching and scratching. Pruritic, discrete nodules often begin in the hair follicles and when scratched, form an excoriated, flattened top, followed by a hard crust. Treatments are usually topical and include glucocorticoids, topical vitamin D3, and capsaicin. Thalidomide and cyclosporins have also been used. Treatment response is variable and lesions are slow to heal, forming hyper-pigmented scars. Confusion with

MD is understandable as the two diseases share many similarities. In fact, there is a dermatology professor who lectures that what MD patients actually have is prurigo nodularis. However, in contrast to biopsies of Morgellons lesions, biopsies of prurigo nodularis lesions reveal eosinophilia and do not contain the filaments diagnostic of MD.

Impetigo

When insect bites or other itchy lesions are scratched, there is a risk of setting up an infection in the open wound by the resident skin bacteria, *Streptococcus pyogenes* or *Staphylococcus aureus*. The infection, called impetigo, is more likely to occur when the skin or nails are dirty and thus is more commonly seen in children. Victims have excoriated lesions with crusty yellow scabs. In contrast to MD lesions, impetigo lesions do not contain filaments and the lesions will often heal with the application of a topical antibiotic that targets *Staphylococcus aureus*, the predominant cause of impetigo. The bacteria that cause impetigo have not been found in the lesions of MD patients and the MD lesions do not heal when a topical antibiotic is applied.

Summary

In summary, the factor that differentiates Morgellons disease from all of these other skin conditions in the differential is the presence of filaments under and protruding from the skin. This particular feature of MD is the disease's unique, identifying factor. That is why a skin examination with lighted 60x to 100x magnification is crucial because to miss the filaments is to miss the disease. But how do you diagnose a disease that doesn't exist in medical textbooks and has no known cause and therefore no reliable lab tests for diagnosis? The following chapter provides insight into this challenge.

DIAGNOSTIC CRITERIA

Clinical Case Definition

Diagnosis of a disease without a known cause or valid diagnostic test requires a clinical case definition in order to assist clinicians inexperienced with the disease in validating the presenting patient's concerns. A clinical case definition is also required to determine who qualifies as a "case" for purposes of epidemiological inclusion. Furthermore, formulating a clinical case definition is a required first step for clinically based research to ensure that patients being studied are a homogenous group. In the absence of a diagnostic test, the current understanding of Morgellons disease is based primarily on the frequency and consistency of the symptoms that are characteristic of its sufferers.

Clinical case definitions of diseases are traditionally based upon a list of symptoms and physical abnormalities that are most commonly seen in the disease's sufferers. The list is formulated with the consensus of the health care providers who have the most experience with the disease.

The Morgellons Research Foundation established a draft case definition for MD in 2007 that included the following 3 criteria:

1. Skin lesions, both spontaneous and self-generated with intense itching. Lesions progress to open wounds that heal abnormally or incompletely.
2. Crawling sensations both within and on the skin surface. Often conceptualized as "bugs moving, stinging or biting" intermittently. May involve scalp, nostrils, ear canal, mouth, head and body hair.
3. Fatigue significant enough to interfere with activities of daily living.

166

This preliminary clinical case definition was inadequate. The distinctive and diagnostic feature of Morgellons disease is the presence of microscopic, subcutaneous filaments that work their way through the skin causing itching, pain, and open lesions. The filaments were not even mentioned in this early case definition. I propose that the clinical case definition simply be that patients must have filaments under and protruding from the skin, since this is the distinguishing feature. Patients with MD present with many different symptoms and not every case is the same. The presence of the filaments is common to all of them and crucial to an MD diagnosis.

Laboratory Analysis

Patients often ask why I do not send a biopsy of one of their lesions to a commercial laboratory for diagnosis. Skin biopsies of MD patient lesions analyzed by commercial laboratories have revealed non-specific pathology or an inflammatory process with no observable pathogens. Unfortunately, commercial laboratories look for what is already known and use a basic algorithm to narrow down pathogens into known categories. When a new pathogen appears on the scene, commercial laboratory pathologists are not oriented towards or equipped to discover new organisms. Only research laboratories do this and research laboratories cannot legally diagnose patients.

Biopsies that are performed on MD patients have included fibrous material projecting from inflamed epidermal tissue which laboratories label as "textile fibers". However, a more thorough analysis of the filaments, performed by the Federal Bureau of Investigation forensics lab, revealed that MD filaments do not resemble textiles or any other man-made substance. Furthermore, as we will discuss in a later chapter, research by Middelveen et al shows the filaments to be made of the inert, organic materials, collagen and keratin.

If a clinician were to send MD patient scabs or tissue to a commercial laboratory, it would be most helpful to order examinations using silver nitrate-based histochemical stains like *Dieterle* or *Warthin-Starry*. This is a straightforward technique for pathologists and would allow spirochetes to be visualized in the samples. Although the type of spirochete cannot be differentiated using these stains, at least the presence of a bacteria not normally found in the skin could sway a clinician against a delusional diagnosis!

Summary

If all health care providers were to utilize a systematic, non-judgmental approach with each and every patient, despite the patient's appearance, behavior, race, color, creed, or symptom oddity, the risk of neglecting or misdiagnosing patients would be greatly reduced. It has been my experience that patients with rare and unusual symptoms report that the lack of reassurance and validation they experience is as painful as is the disease itself. Documenting the subjective symptoms of Morgellons disease patients and taking them seriously will enable sufferers of the disease to have a voice, to feel respected and validated, to experience hope, and to contribute towards their ultimate validation – the legitimization of their disease.

In summary, diagnosis of Morgellons disease involves:

1. The practitioner having an open mind and taking the time to investigate
2. Validating the patient's concerns and committing to help
3. Ruling out the conditions in the differential
4. The patient reporting classic symptoms of MD (as described in detail earlier)
5. The practitioner seeing filaments, with the assistance of lighted magnification, either protruding from the patient's skin or just underneath the outer layer of skin.

If a patient does not have filaments, they do not have Morgellons disease. Unfortunately, many patients and their health care providers do not take the time to carefully examine the skin with lighted magnification and, when they do, they lack the confidence and experience to differentiate what they are seeing. The next chapter explains how to examine the skin of an MD patient. Expensive equipment is not necessary; patience and perseverance are the keys.

SEEING IS BELIEVING

When I first started examining patients with MD I would break out in a cold sweat and feel my pulse rise and the hair on the back of my neck stand up. There are certain things you are not supposed to see coming out of a human body and all of a sudden I was seeing the strangest things, making me question my sanity. In fact, in my early years of examining MD patients, I would always call in a colleague to verify that I was seeing what I thought I was seeing.

A Confusing Picture – at First

Rarely are the filaments of Morgellons patients visible with the naked eye. Dermatologists usually carry a dermatoscope in their pockets but these scopes are typically only capable of 10-14x magnification. A magnifier that is at least 30x but preferably 60x to 100x is required and it should be lighted to help with visualization. Having a UV (ultraviolet) light on the magnifier is particularly helpful in differentiating filaments from human hairs because MD fibers fluoresce under UV light.

With a little experience, it becomes easier to see the difference between hairs and filaments without a UV light. Hairs come to a fine point at the end whereas the filaments have a tubular or ribbon-like look to them. The filaments are usually smaller in diameter than hairs and are often seen intertwined. The dermatologists who have looked at Morgellons skin at 60 - 100x magnification report that it is easy to distinguish between the two once the filaments have been seen a few times.

Accidental contaminants from the environment can sometimes stick to any sort of open wound. It is not uncommon to find some actual textile from clothing and/or dust contaminant from the air in the lesions of MD patients. This can be confusing to health care providers and researchers at first. However, once they see the unique patterns of Morgellons filaments, they are able to easily distinguish the difference. Dermatologists, who are used to seeing environmental contaminants embedded in skin lesions, say that it is not difficult to distinguish MD filaments from accidentally attached debris.

After years of searching for filaments in MD patients and trying many different types of magnifiers to achieve this, both the nurses with the CEHMDF and I have narrowed the choices down to two options – one that is very inexpensive and one that is not. The latter is not necessary but is helpful if you are a health care provider wanting to document your findings. I will discuss these two options here.

The Magnifier Everyone Can Afford

The inexpensive but nonetheless effective way to look for filaments in and on the skin is a gadget that you can find on eBay. This tiny hand-held 60x lighted microscope is easy to hold and work with and even has a UV light. These little scopes are sold new on eBay and I last saw them there for $3.27 each with free shipping, which is affordable by anyone's standards. The price varies and is sometimes as low as $2.09. When the battery dies it costs about the same to order a new magnifier as it does to replace the battery, so order several at once!

The exact name of the item for your search on eBay is "Jewelry Loupe LED Magnifier 60X Mini Microscope Pocket Magnifying Glass UV Light". One drawback of this low-cost magnifier is that you cannot show exactly what you are seeing to anyone else and you cannot photograph what you see for documentation. Another potential drawback is that the magnifier ships from China and so you may wait 4 to 6 weeks for delivery.

The Proscope

The more expensive yet unrivaled method for finding and documenting skin filaments is the

ProScope HR or HR2 by *Bodelin Technologies*. Placing this handheld device on the skin allows everyone in the room to see the same image as it displays on the computer screen. At any point in time, a photograph may be taken of an image to save to the computer's hard drive. This feature makes it easy for patients to send digital photographs to their doctors and for doctors to transport images into the patient's medical record. Costs at this writing are $400+ for the HR and $700+ for the HR2, which has higher resolution and therefore clearer photographs.

There are other options besides the *Proscope* that are very similar in function. I have not taken the time to compare them so I am not familiar with the pros and cons of each. You may want to look around on the Internet for what you can find. I can only speak for the ProScope having successfully used that one. I have no financial interest in any of these products.

The most important thing for practitioners to do is to take the time to look. The filaments are often not seen on the first try and many different parts of the body may need to be examined. It is unfortunate that MD patients present themselves in such a way to health care providers that their symptoms are often discounted and an exam of the skin is never conducted. A later chapter discusses this unfortunate situation.

Part Two

Demographics

"Not everything that counts can be counted and not everything that can be counted counts.

— Albert Einstein

PREDISPOSITIONS TO MORGELLONS DISEASE

Predispositions to Morgellons disease, based on my clinical observations and the results of my descriptive study, are a compromised immune system, cigarette smoking, and Lyme and/or other tickborne diseases. Psychopathology, contrary to the opinion of many clinicians, is NOT a predisposition to MD. A discussion of these disease predispositions follows.

Compromised Immune System

My experience has shown that when patients begin to develop symptoms of MD they usually have immune systems that are suppressed due to chronic infection (either overt or indolent), toxic exposures (physical or psychological) and/or immunosuppressant therapy. Patients with acquired immune deficiency syndrome (AIDS), autoimmune diseases such as systemic lupus erythematosus or rheumatoid arthritis, organ transplants, hepatitis C, or other viral or bacterial illnesses are among those who have come to my office with classic MD symptoms. There are also patients who unknowingly live in a mold-infested home, are exposed to toxins at work or suffer from a disabling psychosocial environment such as PTSD (post traumatic stress disorder) or living with an abusive spouse. These immune challenges are often not immediately obvious until evaluation of the skin symptoms occurs, at which time the thorough clinician should tirelessly investigate to detect the root causes of the patient's debilitated condition.

Cigarette Smoking and Compromised Skin Immunity

There is strong evidence in numerous studies that smoking cigarettes is associated *negatively* with many skin conditions, including poor wound healing, premature aging of the skin, squamous cell carcinoma, psoriasis, hair loss, oral cancers, and other oral conditions. Therefore, patients who smoke cigarettes are at increased risk for numerous skin conditions and skin manifestations of disease and/or will experience delayed healing time for these infections. Of interest is that my research findings revealed that 39% of my MD subjects were smokers as opposed to the 17.8% expected for a similarly matched group in the population at large.

Relationship to Tickborne diseases

Many patients with Morgellons disease have positive blood tests for tickborne pathogens including *Borrelia burgdorferi* (*Bb*), the spirochetal bacteria that cause Lyme disease. Furthermore, *Bb* was cultured from the skin lesions of 24 of 25 Morgellons patients sampled in the research of Middelveen et al. Other tickborne diseases in Morgellons patients, diagnosed by blood tests, include infection with the parasites *Babesia microti* or *Babesia duncani*, the rickettsiae *Ehrlichia chafeensis* or *Anaplasma phagocytophylum*, and the bacteria *Bartonella quintana* or *Bartonella henselae*. Since ticks are known to harbor fungi, parasites, viruses, rickettsiae, and numerous other types of human and plant pathogens, the pathogen that causes MD may prove to be another in a growing list of tickborne co-infections or it may be a dermatological manifestation of Lyme or one of the other tickborne diseases. More about the relationship of MD with tickborne diseases is discussed in a later chapter.

PRECIPITATING FACTORS FOR MORGELLONS DISEASE

Various precipitating events were reported in my study group of 122 MD patients but in many cases (24%), subjects were unaware of an association of any event with the initiation of their symptoms. The most frequent precipitating events were, in descending order of frequency: an infestation of biting insects such as lice or fleas; a recent visit to a 3rd world country; a splinter, thorn, or dirty cut; working in dirt or exposure to dirty water. Of note is that most involve exposure to unclean situations.

Anecdotally, here are some of the reports I have heard from patients in regard to what occurred shortly before their Morgellons symptoms began.

1. A squirrel infestation after the home was vacated for a month while on vacation
2. Cleaning bird nests out of an attic

3. Moving into an apartment that was infested with fleas (this is a common one)
4. Swimming in the Ganges River in India
5. Working in the garden with fertilizer without wearing gloves
6. Wading through a dirty pond
7. Being stuck by a splinter, cactus or rose thorn while working outside

The fact that patients tend to have been exposed to dirty situations before initiation of their symptoms is another factor raising suspicion that MD has a pathogenic rather than a psychosomatic cause.

EPIDEMIOLOGY AND DEMOGRAPHICS

Much of the early epidemiology and other characteristics of Morgellons disease was based on the data collected by the MRF on their now-defunct website where sufferers were invited to register and complete a questionnaire. The total number of registrants on the MRF website at the time it shut down in early 2012 was over 20,000, which is believed to be a small fraction of the actual number of cases of MD. In 2012 the OSU Center for Health Sciences Morgellons Disease Registration Database became the new online self-reporting site for MD patients. The OSU registration database went off-line in 2015 at which time it had over 12,000 registrants. The CEHMDF is in the process of setting up a new registration website for MD patients.

Inherent selection bias exists in internet-based data collection systems such as the MRF and OSU websites. Users of Internet resources may over-represent a well–educated, middle to upper-middle class faction of society. This potentially biased representation of the population could skew the demographic data. Furthermore, in a self-report, disease-registration system, there is the risk that participants who register do not actually have the disease or that their symptoms are exaggerated to fit what the registrant feels is appropriate to the disease.

In 2012, California, Texas, and Florida were the states with the highest self-reported incidence of Morgellons disease based on both the MRF website and my published descriptive study. This finding appears to be independent of the fact that these are the states with the largest number of inhabitants because the *percentage* of the population infected was also higher in these states. For example, California contains 12% of the US population, but 26% of the registrants on the MRF web site were from California (MRF). Likewise, Texas makes up 7.4% of the US population, but 10% of MD registrants were from Texas. In contrast, New York includes 6.7% of the US population, but only 2.3% of reported Morgellons cases. The OSU website statistics are quite different, with Oklahoma, Nevada, and Oregon, being the 3 states with the highest per capita incidence, based on self-reported data. It is not clear why there is such a discrepancy in the findings of the OSU database.

According to the MRF database, an approximately equal number of males and females registered claiming to be affected with the symptoms of MD. The OSU website reported two thirds of registrants identifying as female and one third as male. On both sites, there were registrants in all age groups and from all walks of life: the rich and the poor, professionals and manual laborers, people with basic educations and with those with advanced degrees.

In my descriptive study, more female than male patients had Morgellons disease (84.4% female) based upon my in-office examination of their skin. In fact, my sample group consisted primarily of middle-aged Caucasians. My clinic does not accept any form of insurance and the cash-only visits may have biased towards an upper-middle-class socioeconomic group. This, in turn, may have predisposed toward Caucasian race and older, more economically stable subjects. There are many diseases that appear to be predominantly female but this may be due to the fact that females present more often for medical care, a phenomenon that is thought to skew the statistics of many illnesses known to be predominantly female, including chronic fatigue syndrome, fibromyalgia, lupus, rheumatoid arthritis, multiple sclerosis, Sjogren's syndrome, migraines, gallbladder disease, and irritable bowel syndrome.

In my Morgellons disease study cohort the average age was 47.8 years with a range of 22 to 85. However, I have treated children as young as 9 months old with MD and as old as 88. Professions of patients in my study group were varied and did not seem to suggest any particular high-risk profession other than those who worked outside and were exposed to dirt. Earlier statistics based on the MRF website self-reporting tool showed a predominance of patients who were employed as nurses. The findings of my study did not bear this out. There may have been more respondents to the MRF self-report tool who were nurses and therefore aware of the importance of completing the form in order to make their voices heard.

It is now evident that Morgellons disease is seen all over the world. We have heard reports from all over the United States, South and Central America, Canada, Africa, Asia, Russia, Australia, New Zealand, Malaysia and all of Europe. I have been asked to speak on the topic at medical conferences in The Netherlands, Belgium, Austria, England, Finland, and Germany. When I do speak for these European conferences the doctors who attend are urgently searching for answers, knowing that their MD patients are experiencing a legitimate disease. There are still skeptics in these other countries, but the fact that many doctors understand that MD is a grave physiological disease and want to learn more about it provides hope that other health care providers may soon see the light.

Part Three

The Internet: Friend & Foe

*"Don't believe everything you hear.
There are always 3 sides to every story –
Yours, theirs and the truth".*

— Unknown

JUMPING TO CONCLUSIONS: WHY MORGELLONS PATIENTS ARE OFTEN THEIR OWN WORST ENEMIES

In an earlier chapter, we learned that the Swedish neurologist, Dr. Ekbom, proposed that patients who have been diagnosed with delusions of parasitosis are not delusional: they are simply inept at describing the very real sensations they are experiencing. Unfortunately, in an attempt to explain their unusual symptoms, Morgellons patients often use descriptions that lead to prejudicial treatment by clinicians, who automatically assume they have a mental illness.

Examples of typical patient expressions are: "parasites have taken over my belly", "there are cocoons in my hair", "tiny shrimp come out of my skin", "my hair moves and has a life of its own", or "the skin you see on me is not really my skin." I am constantly coaching my MD patients to list their symptoms in a more descriptive way when speaking to health care providers without giving names to the things that come out of their bodies. So instead of "shrimp come out of my skin", I advise them to say, "tiny, pink, firm crescent-shaped tissue comes out of my skin". Unfortunately, patients can be their own worst enemies when not describing their symptoms accurately.

Due to an abundance of medical information (and misinformation) on the Internet, there is a tendency for patients with all sorts of symptoms to self-diagnose. However, it is best for a patient to list and describe symptoms rather than provide diagnoses to their health care provider. Clinicians are trained to know the differential diagnosis for each and every symptom and patients who are good "historians" (able to report the history and description of their symptoms in detail) are more likely to be taken seriously than those who come in with a firm belief in a certain diagnosis.

The Parasite Confusion

Morgellons patients often present to health care providers having diagnosed themselves with a parasitic infection. Patients tend to be confused about the topic of parasites and understandably so. Let us briefly review the topic in order to help clear up some of the misunderstandings.

In the broadest sense of the term, a parasite is an organism that depends on another organism for its survival, at the expense of the organism that it is dependent upon. So, the term parasite does not specify a particular type of pathogen. There are 3 main categories of parasites that cause disease in humans: 1. Helminths, 2. Ectoparasites and, 3. Protozoa. These different categories could not be more dissimilar. The fact that they all fall under the term "parasite" shows what a broad category the word represents and why there is so much confusion surrounding it.

Helminths are commonly known as worms. Examples of worms that are parasites to humans are flatworms (flukes and tapeworms), thorny headed worms and round worms (aka nematodes such as filariae). Many MD patients believe that they are infested with a parasitic worm (a helminth) due to the fact that the filaments are long and thin, look similar to a worm, and appear to move. The filaments, however, as was reviewed in a previous chapter, have been proven **not** to be worms, so patients should not jump to this conclusion when describing their symptoms to their health care provider.

Ectoparasites are arthropods and include lice, mites, bed bugs and other small biting insects. Ectoparasites have an exoskeleton (external skeleton), a segmented body and jointed appendages. The term "infestation" is used when referring to an ectoparasitic infection. There are many MD patients that are convinced that an ectoparasite is the cause of their symptoms. The biting sensations that they experience make them feel as though they are infested with tiny biting bugs so it is not difficult to understand why MD patients would jump to this conclusion. However, ectoparasites have been ruled out as the cause of Morgellons disease. Therefore, MD patients should **not** tell clinicians that they are infested with "bugs" because they will likely be treated prejudicially.

Finally, there are the unicellular, protozoan parasites that, unlike the helminths and ectoparasites, are not visible to the naked eye. Microscopic protozoan parasites cause diseases like malaria, amoebic dysentery, giardia, babesiosis, leishmaniasis, and toxoplasmosis. We do not yet know for certain whether protozoa cause MD although none have been isolated so far in the research. However, Morgellons patients who tell clinicians that they have parasites are usually thinking of helminths or ectoparasites, rather than protozoa.

Just to confuse the topic even more, certain bacteria can also be parasites and, like protozoa, are microscopic. If a bacterium lives in the human body and uses the human host in order to thrive and multiply so that the bacterium can then go on to infect others, it is said to be parasitic. Examples of human diseases caused by parasitic bacteria include salmonella, syphilis, Lyme disease, gonorrhea, cholera, small pox and Bubonic plague. Just to be clear, **not all bacteria are parasites!**

The cause of MD may very well prove to be a parasitic bacterium. But bacteria are microscopic and, once again, when MD patients state that they have parasites, they are usually referring to the visible-to-the-naked-eye helminths or ectoparasites (both of which we **know** do not cause Morgellons disease) rather than the microscopic protozoa or parasitic bacteria. Even health care providers, upon hearing the word "parasite", have a tendency to think primarily of helminths or ectoparasites. This is why it behooves patients not to use the word in order to avoid confusion or prejudicial treatment by clinicians.

In summary, Morgellons disease is **not** caused by a helminth or by an ectoparasitic infestation and when patients use the word parasite, they are usually referring to one of these two categories. Unfortunately, patients can be their own worst enemies when they describe their symptoms in an inaccurate way or jump to conclusions about what is causing their symptoms. Health care providers tend to discount these patients and, unfortunately, jump to the conclusion that these same patients are mentally unstable.

DISPELLING THE MYTHS

As mentioned in the previous chapter, the Internet is awash with diverse speculations about the cause of Morgellons disease. It is understandable that sufferers would spend many hours online researching the cause of their symptoms. Unfortunately, they are often exposed to misinformation. In this chapter, I will list the most commonly held myths promulgated on the Internet about Morgellons disease and how they have been disproven over the years.

Myth #1. Morgellons disease is caused by Springtails (Collembola)

The earliest research on Morgellons disease was in 2004 when the insect Collembola was suggested as the possible causative pathogen in a paper by Altschuler et al, published in the *Journal of the New York Entomological Society*. The authors of the paper had found collembola in the skin scrapings of 20 patients previously diagnosed with DOP. However, further research by 3 different researchers, Wymore, Middelveen, and Sapi, has not corroborated this finding. If Springtails were the cause of MD they would be fairly easy to identify. Plus, this type of infestation would not explain the filaments, which are the distinctive feature of Morgellons disease.

Myth #2. Morgellons disease is caused by a GMO (genetically modified organism)

The first Food & Drug Administration (FDA)-approved GMO appeared on the market in 1982. It was Humulin, a type of insulin for diabetics, genetically engineered by *E.coli* bacteria. Over the years since then, tobacco and food crops have been genetically modified with the goal of making crops more resistant to weeds and insects and promoting longer shelf life of foods.

To quote the 1970's Chiffon margarine commercial, "It's not nice to fool Mother Nature."

Genetically modified foods are a great concern for our health and welfare since the body reacts with inflammation to ingested substances not recognized as pure food.

It is tempting to believe that the pathogen causing MD could be a GMO. There has been no proof for or against this theory. But the main argument refuting this position is that MD has been around **much** longer than GMOs have, as explained earlier in this book. GMOs are a relatively new phenomenon. Morgellons disease is not.

Myth #3. Morgellons disease is caused by something distributed by chemtrails

According to the chemtrail theory, long-lasting trails behind high-flying aircraft contain aerosolized particulate used for geo-engineering, weather-modification and military purposes. It is proposed that this spray causes the general population to be over - exposed to aluminum oxide and other toxic metals and chemicals. Heavy metal toxicity is known to burden the immune system making those exposed more vulnerable to all kinds of disease. Furthermore, studies have shown specifically that Lyme patients with a heavy aluminum load have more difficult-to-treat infections.

So, if in fact there were a relationship between MD and chemtrails, it would simply be that those with immune systems burdened by metal toxicity are more susceptible to it or to any other disease. Furthermore, we run into the same conundrum that we face with the GMO theory: the chemtrail discussion started appearing on the Internet in the 1990s. Morgellons disease has been around much longer than that. In summary, chemtrails and GMO's do **not cause** Morgellons disease. However, they **may** make certain susceptible individuals more vulnerable to any number of immune challenges, one of which could be Morgellons disease.

Myth #4. Morgellons disease is due to mold exposure

Exposure to toxic molds also places an extra burden on the immune system, making those who are exposed more susceptible to all kinds of infections and inflammatory conditions, particularly if they are genetically predisposed to have difficulty clearing mold toxins. The pioneering work of Richard Shoemaker, M.D. taught us that mold toxicity and Lyme disease are a particularly ominous combination with exposure to both simultaneously making treatment of either more challenging. **Mold exposure does not cause Morgellons disease** but it can certainly make someone more likely to become ill with it or have a more severe, difficult-to-treat case.

Myth #5. Morgellons filaments are filarial worms or another thread-like worm

A large number of patients continue to be adamant that MD is caused by thread-like worms called microfilariae. Although filariasis is typically spread by mosquito bites, it has been known for quite some time that filarial worms are also in the tick gut along with dozens of other types of pathogens. Therefore, proponents of this theory believe that the microfilaria infection that they purport causes MD is a tickborne co-infection and therein lies the connection to Lyme disease.

Patients will often find earlier writings of the late Dr. William Harvey when he served on the MRF Board of Directors in which he proposed that worms might cause MD. Recent reports that Dr. Alan McDonald has discovered filarial worms along with Lyme spirochetes in the brains of Alzheimer's patients has caused many Morgellons patients to fear that the fibers of MD are actually filarial worms, just like those found by Dr. McDonald in human brains (photographs of the two do look very similar).

Morgellons disease may very well be caused by a pathogen that is parasitic in nature (requires a host in order to survive). However, parasitic worms do **not** cause MD. The filaments are inanimate objects made of collagen and keratin, normal proteins of the human body. The filaments are **not** filariasis or any other thread-like worm. The fact that the filaments occasionally appear to move does not mean that they are alive – the movement is most likely due to an electrostatic charge.

Myth # 6. Morgellons disease is associated with the fungus Glomus-versiforme or caused by some other fungus

It has been tempting from the start to label MD a fungal infection. The filaments fluoresce under ultraviolet light, which is true of fungi. The network of filaments under the skin branch out in different directions similar to the branching of fungi. Moreover, some MD patients are even helped by antifungals. However, all of the research performed so far has not been able to detect any kind of fungal pathogen.

There are many patients who become downright angry upon hearing that the responsible pathogen for MD is not fungal. They remain quite sure that it is because in their particular case antifungals helped them to heal. I am quite sure that I have treated more Morgellons patients than anyone else in the world and I can guarantee that the vast majority of MD patients do **not** respond to antifungals.

I suspect that in the few cases where patients appear to have derived benefit from antifungals it is because they had an indolent, co-existing, fungal infection and by removing the burden of this underlying infection the immune system was able to battle the pathogen responsible for MD.

Myth #7. Morgellons disease is caused by allergenic dental materials

There is a parasitologist who believes that

MD results when dental amalgams that are incompatible with the human body cause inflammation and neurotoxicity. The resultant damage to the nerves purportedly causes a type of neuropathy that leads patients to believe that there are bugs crawling on or under their skin. This theory posits that when the lymphatic system tries to eliminate these toxins, sores break out on the skin that attract other organisms to adhere to them, like fungal spores which cause growths.

There has been much written about metal amalgams in the mouth purporting that they impair functioning of the immune system due to their toxic nature. So, for those with metals in their mouths, there may be an increased susceptibility to any number of chronic, fatiguing illnesses – possibly even Morgellons disease. But the sensations that Morgellons patients experience are not merely neuropathies. There is a reason for the discomfort – there are filaments growing under the skin. These filaments are deeply embedded and not caused by something adhering to the open lesions. Furthermore, as stated previously, research has shown no fungal component to Morgellons disease.

Myth #8. Morgellons disease is caused by an agrobacterium, a bacterium that infects trees

The idea that agrobacteria might be the pathogens responsible for MD was proposed by Raphael Stricker, MD in 2007 and research looking for agrobacteria in Morgellons lesions was performed by Vitaly Citovsky, Ph.D. at the State University of New York at Stoney Brook that same year. One early study by the MRF had proposed that MD filaments were composed of cellulose, making the idea that a plant pathogen might be the culprit an enticing idea to investigate. In Dr. Citovsky's preliminary study, all 7 of my Morgellons patients whose skin biopsies were analyzed revealed evidence of infection with *Agrobacteria*, whereas biopsies of 7 control subjects did not.

This finding could never be duplicated in other laboratories and contamination was suspected in Dr. Citovsky's lab since he specialized in studying agrobacteria. Furthermore, it has been discovered that filaments are composed of keratin and collagen, rather than cellulose, making the agrobacterium idea highly unlikely. Therefore, this theory was never substantiated and was abandoned. Many people today read the old information on this theory and incorrectly conclude that agrobacteria are the cause of MD.

Myth #9. Morgellons disease is caused by a Dermacentor or other type of barely-visible mite.

Most Dermacentor mites are not seen by the naked eye. Many Morgellons patients are convinced that they have mites because the sensations they experience feel like bites. People certainly can have mite infestations but this is an entirely different issue than Morgellons disease. Again, it comes back down to the filaments and the fact that if mites were the culprits they would be able to be seen with magnification.

Myth #10. Morgellons disease is caused by myiasis (infestation of fly larvae) of a very tiny fly

Myiasis is caused by an infestation with larvae of the human botfly or tambu fly and is most commonly found in tropical areas. The larvae (maggots) can be seen without magnification, being 1 to 2 cm long and growing to the size of a goose egg. The idea that there may be a myiasis infection caused by very tiny maggots of very tiny flies is a theory that some have come up with to explain Morgellons disease, a theory that very many patients firmly adhere to. So far, research has not identified any type of insect larva in the skin of MD patients. Plus, once again, there is the issue of the filaments, which have no logical explanation in a myiasis theory of MD.

Myth #11 Morgellons is a man-made disease, developed for biowarfare that has accidentally (or purposely?) been released into the population at large.

There has been no evidence that substantiates or disproves this theory. This seems unlikely to me but only time will tell.

BEWARE OF FALSE PROPHETS

As discussed in the previous chapter, there are numerous unscientific theories and rumors regarding the cause of Morgellons disease. Patients are exposed to these ideas when they search the Internet trying to understand what is happening to them. Even more unscrupulous than these purveyors of unscientific information are the "snake oil salesmen" who lead patients down blind alleys and rob them of their finances. Any desperate, uninformed group of downtrodden people easily falls prey to entrepreneurs without scruples who see a great opportunity to take advantage of their vulnerability and misfortune. There have been all sorts of internal and external treatments marketed to MD patients with the promise of making them whole again. Desperate people are willing to try any treatment if there isvthe slightest chance of a cure.

Patients should be wary of any product salesman who says he can heal them. Many of these sales people will actually say that they have TREATED thousands of MD patients. Salesmen do not treat patients. They sell products and will use any method that works to make a sale. If a sales person says that every MD patient who has bought their product has improved, remember that they do not have the long term follow up with patients that a health care provider does. They are not interpreting lab results, seeing and examining patients on a regular basis, and following patient symptoms in detail. You can have confidence in a treatment if a health care provider who has treated many MD patients and tried numerous different treatment methods recommends it. You can be particularly reassured if they have no financial incentive to endorse it.

Over the years, sales representatives for products marketed to MD patients have approached me about endorsing their products or selling them in my office. When they tell me how miraculously effective their products are, I ask if they have patient follow-up statistics. Usually, their follow up with patients has been no more than 2 weeks after the patient has started their product. I have noticed that every topical product an MD patient tries works well for 2 weeks and then stops working. The same is true for most "natural" antimicrobials. So, unless there is long-term follow-up showing continued improvement over many months, I have no interest in the product. Petroleum jelly works well as a topical treatment for Morgellons patients too – for 2 weeks – and is very inexpensive and easy to come by!

Part Four

Towards Understanding

"Nothing in life is to be feared, it is only to be understood. Now is the time to understand more, so that we may fear less."

— Marie Curie

RESEARCHING A NEW DISEASE

Research on the cause of a new disease involves a considerable amount of time and money. Expenses include salaries of the researchers, use and maintenance of a laboratory facility, lab equipment and supplies such as vials and reagents. Most people are unaware of the expensive involved in acquiring lab supplies and the hundreds of professional staff hours that go into taking just a small step forward in research.

Morgellons disease is still considered a non-disease by most of the medical community. In other words, it is believed to be a psychoneurotic condition rather than one with an underlying physical cause. For this reason, obtaining funding from the usual sources is virtually impossible. About 10 years ago a few colleagues and I applied to the National Institutes of Health for grant money to study the disease and the reply was "We do not provide funding for research on diseases that do not exist".

So we are caught in a Catch-22. We cannot prove the disease's existence as a true medical condition until we obtain funding for research and we cannot obtain funding for research until we prove that the disease is a true medical condition. The research that **has** been performed has been thanks to private donations and the valuable non-paid time of interested professional researchers.

This chapter will review the research on Morgellons disease that has been conducted so far. There will be some scientific terms that will be difficult for the lay reader to understand but everyone can benefit from knowing that there are scientists and clinicians who are working diligently to put together the pieces of this diagnostic puzzle. The reality of Morgellons as a physiologic disease is becoming increasingly difficult to refute.

Jenny Haverty

In late 2004, Jenny Haverty, a clinical

microbiologist at Marin General Hospital in Marin County, California, examined filaments from skin samples of 4 different MD patients from the San Francisco Bay area. She found that samples contained clear tubular-shaped filaments; clear, red or black ribbon-like filaments; brown filaments with ladder-like rungs, and smaller filaments that were clear, white, black, red or blue. The red and black filaments did not fluoresce under ultraviolet ("black") light whereas all of the other filaments fluoresced a bright aqua color. Ms. Haverty proposed that the similarities in the filaments of these patients suggested that the causative agent for all 4 cases was epidemiologically the same.

Center for Investigation of Morgellons Disease

Randy S. Wymore, Ph.D., was the first scientist to perform serious research into the causative pathogen of MD at the Center for Investigation of Morgellons Disease established at the Oklahoma State University Center for Health Sciences in Tulsa, Oklahoma in 2005.

Dr. Wymore was the first researcher to ascertain that:

- The filaments are NOT textile or any other manmade substance
- The cause of Morgellons disease is NOT fungal
- Both Collembola and *Stenotrophomonas maltophilia* can be ruled out as possible causative pathogens of Morgellons disease
- The black "specks" that patients complain of and often think are "bugs" are nothing more than fibers wound up in tight balls
- Filaments coil themselves tightly around the hairs of Morgellons disease patients
- In contrast to Dr. Vidal Citovsky's findings, Agrobacteria are not found in biopsies   of Morgellons patients

Dr. Wymore's research continues today. In the Wymore lab, they are using a combination of microbiology and molecular biology strategies to further examine the details of the infective

226

process. In addition to *Bartonella henselae* (the causative pathogen of Bartonellosis or "Cat Scratch Fever"), Dr. Wymore and his team have isolated 3 other bacteria in Morgellons samples collected from a dispersed geographic area. These 3 bacteria are all spirochetes: *Borrelia burgdorferi* (the causative pathogen of Lyme disease), *Treponema denticola* and *Helicobacter pylori* (the last two are discussed below). Spirochetes are bacteria that often live in a coiled shape, a shape that is highly motile and able to penetrate deep into the tissues (much as a corkscrew enters the dense cork at the top of a wine bottle).

T. denticola, a spirochete that is usually associated with periodontal disease, is a genus relative of the Syphilis spirochete (*Treponema pallidum*). *H.pylori*, the other spirochete isolate in MD biopsies by Wymore's team, is most commonly associated with stomach ulcers. Half of the world's population is infected with *H.pylori* but only 10-20% of these people develop an ulcer. Other than stomach ulcers, *H. pylori* have also been associated with autoimmunity, migraines, adrenal fatigue, muscle spasms, tooth decay, allergies, chronic sinusitis, chronic infection, mineral depletion (from neutralizing stomach acid), liver and gall bladder problems. Clearly, there is more that we need to learn about these two spiral-shaped bacteria and their effects in places other than the mouth and the stomach. Dr. Wymore is in the process of finalizing the confirmation and sequencing of these samples prior to submission of a manuscript for publication.

Georgia Department of Public Health

In 2006, in a response to an outcry from MD patients in Georgia, the Georgia health department initiated a surveillance study of "Unidentified Dermatosis Syndrome (UDS) aka Morgellons Disease". A surveillance database was established to collect epidemiologic information about patients in Georgia with MD symptoms. The study was never completed and results never published because the Center for Disease Control (CDC) in Atlanta stepped in and started investigating the disease on a national level.

However, the Director of the Chemical Hazards Program of the Division of Public Health presented preliminary results of the surveillance study at a Georgia health department meeting in September 2007. Collected data revealed that the male-female ratio of responders was about 50-50, there were no notable precipitating factors to the disease, and the disease had no significant correlation with having outdoor hobbies. The majority of reported cases were in the northern half of Georgia and involved recent contact with upturned soils.

No etiological theories were proposed but patients were strongly urged to avoid harsh chemicals to self-treat. According to the Georgia survey, patients had reported using the following caustic chemicals topically in an effort to stop their torturous symptoms: bleach, ammonia, insect spray, dog flea dip, gasoline, kerosene, WD40, Windex, and Lysol.

The CDC Study

The Centers for Disease Control and Prevention (CDC) initiated an investigation into MD in January of 2008 because they had received so many phone calls about the disease and complaints that they were doing nothing about it. For unclear reasons they did not release results until 2012, two years after the study was completed. After spending close to a half million dollars, the CDC was unable to find a pathogen associated with the symptoms and concluded, "No common underlying medical condition or infectious source was identified." Unfortunately, the press took this information and distorted it, presumably for sensational purposes, with headlines claiming that the CDC study found that "Morgellons disease exists only in patients' minds." To be clear, this was not the finding of the

CDC study. **Absence of proof does not equal proof of absence!**

In my opinion, the CDC's commitment to research on this topic was disingenuous. The study was poorly designed and previous research on the topic was ignored and not cited. The researchers looked only for typical skin pathogens and it was already obvious that this endeavor would reveal nothing new. Many Morgellons patients had had their skin biopsies analyzed in commercial laboratories and nothing but "inflammatory changes" had been identified. Furthermore, the CDC's lab analysis methods were far less sophisticated than those being done by volunteer researchers today.

I had offered the CDC my group of pre-screened subjects to use as a study group, thinking that they would be grateful to work with a cohort of patients who all shared the same symptoms and clinical presentation. Rather than taking me up on my offer, the CDC chose to use the Kaiser-Permanente medical group in the San Francisco bay area as their source of subjects. This was perplexing as Kaiser was not even diagnosing MD. There was no consistency to the CDC study group because subjects included anyone who had presented to a Kaiser clinic with feelings of biting, crawling and itching! You cannot have a valid research study without a homogenous group of subjects with clear inclusion and exclusion criteria. Furthermore, since Kaiser had become infamous for not acknowledging MD, my Kaiser patients with MD would not participate in the study because they refused to ever go near a Kaiser clinic again after the mistreatment they had suffered there.

My descriptive study

In 2009 I completed a detailed descriptive study of 122 clinically confirmed cases of Morgellons disease as a part of my doctoral candidacy work. The requirement for inclusion as a study subject was the presence of filaments under the skin, as seen by me in my office. When the results were published in the May 2010 edition of *Clinical, Cosmetic and Investigative Dermatology* it was the first time that a peer-reviewed study published in a medical journal suggested an association between MD and Lyme disease. Of the 122 patients included in the study 97% either tested positive for Lyme disease (53%) or were highly suspect for it, based upon clinical diagnostic criteria (44%). The clinical diagnostic criteria for a Lyme diagnosis were as follows (5 out of the 9 were required):

- History of a Lyme disease diagnosis at any time in the past
- History of a tick bite at any time in the past
- High exposure risk (living in an endemic area, hiking in the woods, etc.)
- Equivalent result on a Lyme Western Blot or presence of bands on the blot that are specific for Bb, despite the fact that the test result was negative

- Positive lab result for any of the tickborne coinfections (Babesia, Bartonella, Ehrlichia, Anaplasma, etc.)
- Below-normal CD57-positive Natural Killer cell count (a blood test marker that has been found to be below normal in Lyme disease patients)
- Above-normal C4a complement protein, a marker that is elevated in chronic inflammatory infections
- Classic Lyme symptoms such as joint pain, exhaustion, cognitive decline, sleep disturbance, muscle aches, etc.
- Flu-like symptoms 4 to 5 days after starting antibiotics signaling a die-off reaction of the spirochetes (called a Jarish-Herxheimer reaction)

It is important to note that 3% of my sample neither tested positive for Lyme disease nor were suspect for it based on the clinical diagnostic criteria stated above. This 3% had absolutely no systemic symptoms along with their MD skin symptoms and did not react to antibiotics the way that Lyme patients are expected to.

However, the 3% (4 subjects) had other challenges suppressing their immune systems, including treatment with high dose prednisone for an autoimmune condition (2), treatment with immune-suppressing, anti-rejection medications for an organ transplant (1) or AIDS (acquired immune deficiency syndrome) (1).

Marianne Middelveen

In 2010, after speaking with a few patients in my waiting room, a Canadian microbiologist named Marianne Middelveen, became fascinated with Morgellons disease and motivated to study the illness on her own time. Ms. Middelveen's background had been in tropical and veterinary diseases and Morgellons reminded her of a spirochetal infection she had known in cows called Bovine Digital Dermatitis (BDD), also known as Mortellaro's Disease and commonly called "hairy heel warts".

In BDD, ulcerative lesions and keratin filaments are found on the hooves of infected cows and collagen/keratin projections are seen under the scabs formed on the lesions. The disease also causes lameness, weight loss and decreased milk production in its bovine hosts. Cheli and Mortellaro first described BDD in Italy in 1974. The disease is a serious economic problem in Europe, affecting as many as 1 in 3 cattle in some European countries. Several bacteria have been purported to be responsible for BDD including a spirochete in the *Treponeme* genus (the genus that includes *Treponema Pallidum*, which is responsible for syphilis).

My association of MD with Lyme disease intrigued Ms. Middelveen. She went on to collaborate with several medical doctors and scientific researchers resulting in 5 papers published between 2011 to 2015 revealing valuable information supporting the legitimacy of the disease as an infectious rather than a psychiatric process. Middelveen and team found

236

Borrelia spirochetes in the skin of every one of 25 MD patients sampled and *Borrelia burgdorferi* specifically (the causative pathogen of Lyme disease) in 24 of the 25, once again raising the interesting association of MD with Lyme disease.

Middelveen's group was also the first to use *Gomori Trichrome* stain to show that MD filaments are composed of the body's own proteins, collagen, and keratin. The following slide (*Image 42*) shows a cross section of a Morgellons

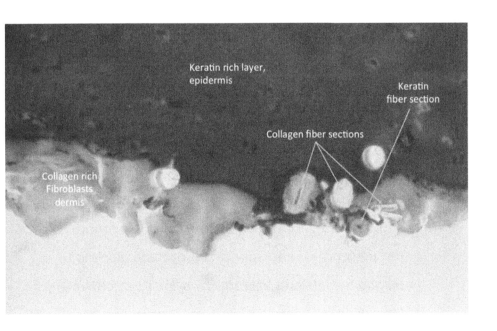

patient's skin stained with *Gomori Trichrome* stain, known to turn keratin red and collagen bluish-green. If you look at the color version of this photograph on gingersavely.com/morgellons-book, you will see the cross sections of keratin filaments (stained red) and collagen filaments (stained bluish-green) just below the keratin rich epidermis (stained red). Photograph used with permission of M. Middelveen.

Eva Sapi, PhD

Eva Sapi, Ph.D. is studying Morgellons disease with the assistance of her graduate students at the University of New Haven, CT, Department of Biology and Environmental Sciences. Using nested PCR (polymerase chain reaction), whole genome direct sequencing with metagenomic analyses, immunohistochemical and in situ methods, Dr. Sapi's group has found the presence of two spirochetal bacteria, *Borrelia burgdorferi (Bb)* and *Helicobacter pylori (H. pylori)* in Morgellons patients' lesions. Sapi's current work is geared towards genotyping the species of *Bb* found in MD lesions and finding genetic commonalities in the MD subjects sampled.

The photograph below (*Image 43*) at 500x magnification reveals the presence of spirochetal structures in MD patients' skin lesions using fluorescent immunohistochemical analyses with *Borrelia* specific monoclonal and polyclonal antibodies. (Used by permission of Dr. Eva Sapi).

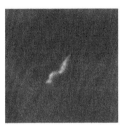 Monoclonal Ab

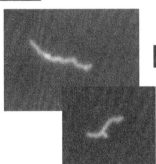 Polyclonal Ab

It is important to note that metagenomic analyses, such as those done at PerkinElmer, Inc. for Dr. Sapi, look for all of the genomes present in a sample. All sorts of microbes may be picked up including those that are unculturable or even unknown. Morgellons researchers have sometimes been accused of finding spirochetes in MD samples because that is what they are looking for. With a metagenomic analysis of a human sample, human DNA will always be present, of course, but there is no way to know what microbial genomes will show up. In other words, it is impossible to examine the sample with any sort of prejudice. Genomes present in the sample will always be a surprise.

Both of the bacteria found by Dr. Sapi, *Bb,* the cause of Lyme disease and *H.pylori,* known for causing stomach ulcers, are spirochetes, the spiral-shaped bacteria that were discussed earlier. Spirochetes prefer not to be in their coiled form because they are more vulnerable this way. Biofilms are protective colonies in which bacteria live. Dr. Sapi's latest data shows that most of the pathogens found in MD lesions are in biofilm form, a form that is well known to be antibiotic resistant. One of the major protectors of biofilm is a sugar called alginate and Sapi's group has found this marker in the biofilms of MD patients. Alginate is gelatinous and may be responsible for the gobs of gelatinous material on the skin reported by MD patients.

Dr. Sapi's recent work shows that *Bb* and *H.pylori* aggregates (dense clusters) and fibers can co-exist in Morgellons disease lesions. *Bb* and *H.pylori* aggregates contain both alginate and amyloid markers such as phospho-tau, suggesting that there are biofilms with amyloid-like changes in the skin samples of Morgellons patients. Phospho-tau in the MD skin suggests that there could be a specific genetic variation in Morgellons patients making the *Bb/H.pylori* infection produce collagen and keratin filaments. This is all conjecture at this point.

Two different epidemiologic studies, one by Peter Mayne, M.D. of Australia (2015) using an Australian cohort and another by Melissa McElroy, FNP of San Francisco, California (2016) using a North American cohort have both revealed that 6% of Lyme patients become victims of MD. This statistic is interesting to me because my guestimate all along, based on my clinical experience, has been about 5-10%. These early epidemiological statistics help answer the question posed by many Lyme disease patients: "Am I doomed to get Morgellons disease because of my Lyme disease?" The connection between Lyme disease and Morgellons disease continues to be compelling but if the spirochete of Lyme disease is the culprit, why do only 6% of Lyme patients get Morgellons disease? Dr. Sapi and her team are exploring this conundrum by looking for genetic variants that MD patients may share in common.

<u>Jyotsna Shah, Ph.D. with IGeneX Laboratories</u>

Since my first involvement with MD in 2003, I had been speaking with Dr. Shah of IGeneX, Inc. Laboratories in Palo Alto, California about the need for research into the connection between Lyme disease and MD and asking for her time and expertise in researching the cause. Dr. Shah was interested and intrigued but, as director of a large laboratory, time constraints precluded her involvement in such a project for many years.

In early 2016 Dr. Shah came on board and donated her time and lab services to a pilot study examining whole blood, serum and skin scraping samples from 10 MD patients using three laboratory techniques: Immunofluorescence Antibody Assay (IFA), Western blot and Polymerase Chain Reaction (PCR). Dr. Shah was interested to find if there were other *Borrelia* species, besides *Borrelia burgdorferi,* (the Lyme pathogen) involved in Morgellons disease. She was particularly interested in the tickborne relapsing fever group.

Tickborne relapsing fever (TBRF) was first recognized just over a hundred years ago. The top symptoms are headaches, muscle aches and chills. The diagnosis is often missed and therefore underreported and new regions of endemicity continue to be identified. Currently, California and Texas are the most highly endemic states in the US. In 1986, Barbour and Hayes associated TBRF with at least 17 different *Borrelia* species. Four species of *Borrelia* that cause TBRF are known in the US: *Borrelia hermsii, Borellia perkerii, Borellia turicate* and *Borrelia miyamotoi. Borrelia myamotoi* is closely related to the other bacteria that cause tickborne relapsing fever but is more distantly related to the *Borrelia* that causes Lyme disease.

In Dr. Shah's pilot study, samples from all 10 MD study subjects were positive for antibodies to *Borrelia* of some kind, either *Bb* (the Lyme disease spirochete) or one of the relapsing fever spirochetes. Relapsing fever *Borrelia* were common to 7 out of 10 samples. Dr. Shah's recommendation, based on her pilot study results, is to perform the following tests on MD patients: Lyme IFA and Western Blot on serum; Lyme PCR on skin scrapings, whole blood and serum; TBRF Western Blot on serum and TBRF PCR on skin scrapings, whole blood and serum.

In summary, many people who have Lyme symptoms but negative test results may be infected with other types of *Borrelia* species that are not being detected on the tests that are currently being used. It has been suggested that the reason that some patients in my previously mentioned descriptive study were negative for Lyme's *Bb* spirochete is that the testing did not include the parameters for other *Borrelia* infections.

Research Continues

In September 2016, a group of European researchers and post-doctoral students met in Leipzig, Germany as the first step in a collaborative effort to research Bovine Digital Dermatitis (BDD - the spirochetal cow disease discussed in an earlier paragraph), its relationship to Morgellons disease and possible effective treatments for both diseases. Present at the meeting was the veterinary researcher who first described BDD in 1974, Professor Carlo Maria Mortellaro of Italy. Also in attendance was Professor Christoph Mülling, Germany's leading expert on BDD and director of the University of Leipzig's department of veterinary research, as well as Carsten Nicolaus, Ph.D., M.D., owner of the Borreliose Centrum clinic in Augsburg, Germany. Dr. Nicolaus, who initiated the collaboration, is an expert on the treatment of tickborne diseases and an advisory board member for the CEHMDF. Obtaining funding should be relatively straightforward since BDD has caused a significant drain on the European economy.

Clearly, more research is needed to unravel the mystery of Morgellons disease. An understanding of the disease's cause and the discovery of an effective treatment is urgently needed since MD patients suffer significant disability. In order to progress with research, the first step is recognition of the problem by the medical community so that funding may be obtained for more expansive and sophisticated studies. This is why the Charles E. Holman foundation and all of us who are on its board of directors and advisory board continue to work to raise awareness and educate medical professionals about the legitimacy of the disease.

Due to a dearth of funding, research has been progressing in baby steps. However, slowly but surely, researchers are making headway. What continues to surface in all investigations is the intriguing association of MD with spirochetal bacteria of various types. What are spirochetes and why are they being mentioned so often in this book? The next chapter will give an overview of this particular phylum of bacteria.

THE MORGELLONS / SPIROCHETE CONNECTION

Spirochetes are long, slender bacteria that are coiled into a helical shape. They look somewhat like a mattress spring, except, of course, they cannot be seen by the naked eye. Some Morgellons patients have told me that they see spirochetes in their eyes or in their lesions. This is impossible considering that spirochetes are so thin they can rarely be seen even under a regular light microscope (darkfield microscopy is required).

An unusual feature of spirochetes is that the flagellum (a "whip-like" appendage that bacteria use for movement) is **internal,** which enables this bacterium to move like a Slinky toy. The ability to alternate between lengthening and recoiling allows spirochetes to enter deeply into tissues. This motion is facilitated by the fact that the width of this bacterium is only a fraction of a micron whereas the length is 5 to 250 microns.

When seen under a microscope, spirochetes appear to wiggle as they undulate across the field of vision.

The most notable genera (plural of genus) of spirochetes are *Treponema, Leptospira,* and *Borrelia.* A close cousin, the genus *Helicobacter* (also helical shaped), is technically not a spirochete but is often included when discussing them because of the many characteristics they share in common. The diseases most commonly associated with these bacteria are Lyme disease, Syphilis, Leptospirosis, Rat Bite Fever, Relapsing Fever, Bejel, Pinta, Yaws and stomach ulcers.

The most often discussed of the *Treponemes* is *Treponema pallidum* that causes Syphilis; the most well-known Borrelia is *Borrelia burgdorferi* that causes Lyme disease; and the most disease-associated of the *Helicobacter* are Helicobacter pylori that cause stomach ulcers. *Treponema, Borrelia,* and *Helicobacter* genera have been mentioned throughout this book. Even in

Ekbom's work nearly a century ago an association with *Treponema pallidum* was noticed in those who were being diagnosed with a disorder known as "parasitophobia", an earlier name for those who we now believe to have Morgellons disease.

Bovine digital dermatitis (BDD), the previously discussed cow disease that shares features with Morgellons disease in humans, is caused in part by a *Treponeme*. Dr. Wymore and his team found 3 different spirochetes in Morgellons lesions: *Treponema denticola, Borrelia burgdorferi* and *Helicobacter pylori*. Dr. Eva Sapi's group discovered the spirochetes *Borrelia burgdorferi* and *Helicobacter pylori* in their biopsies from MD patients. Ms. Middelveen and colleagues have found *Borrelia* spirochetes in 25 out of 25 Morgellons patients sampled. Finally, Dr. Jyotsna Shah has uncovered 2 different species of *Borrelia* spirochetes in the samples she has tested.

Spirochetes are not the only bacteria found in MD patients' biopsies – *Bartonella species*,

251

gram-negative bacteria that are not spirochetes, have been found as well. However, one cannot help but wonder about this striking connection between spirochetes and Morgellons disease. With future research, we will watch the resolution of this puzzle slowly begin to unfold.

Of all of the spirochetes we have discussed so far, *Borrelia burgdoferi (Bb)*, the spirochete responsible for Lyme disease, has surfaced most frequently in correlation with Morgellons disease. In the next chapter we will look at the connection between *Bb* and MD and review the evidence that either supports or refutes the hypothesis that Morgellons disease is a dermatological manifestation of Lyme disease.

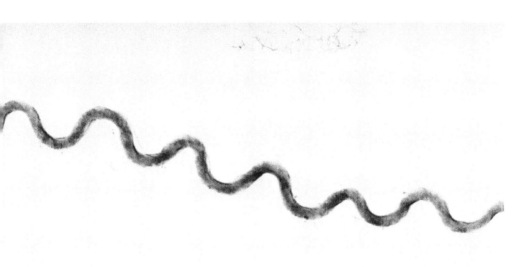

Image 44: Photomicrograph of a spirochete (in this case, Treponema pallidum), by Bill Schwartz, CDC, Courtesy: Public Health Image Library. Public domain.

THE LYME DISEASE CONNECTION

What is Lyme disease?

Lyme disease is a bacterial infection caused by the spirochete, *Borrelia burgdorferi* (*Bb*). It was named for the town of Lyme, Connecticut, where an outbreak occurred in 1975. Lyme disease is almost always spread through the bite of a tick although other biting insects may also be culprits. When it is diagnosed promptly it is not a particularly difficult infection to treat. The problem is that Lyme disease is usually missed in its early, more treatable stage.

Fifty percent of patients do not get the characteristic and diagnostic "bull's eye rash" and at least that many do not even recall a tick bite. The nymphal tick that spreads the disease is the size of a poppy seed and very easy to miss when on dark skin or a hairy part of the body. Early symptoms are non-specific and often confused with a virus. Even if a health care practitioner does think to test for Lyme disease, current tests have an unacceptably large percentage of false negatives.

When missed in its acute stage, Lyme disease can quickly disseminate throughout the entire body wreaking havoc with every body system. It masquerades as many different conditions so the disseminated, persistent form of the disease is even more confusing to diagnose than the acute form. When I first evaluate a Morgellons patient they often say something like, "I've heard about the association between Morgellons disease and Lyme disease, but there is no way I could have Lyme disease. I would know it if I did, right?" Actually, the answer is no. Most people with persistent Lyme disease do NOT know they have it and are misdiagnosed with labels like Fibromyalgia, Chronic Fatigue Syndrome, Lupus, Multiple Sclerosis, Early Onset Alzheimer's, Rheumatoid Arthritis, Migraines, Irritable Bowel Syndrome, Interstitial Cystitis, and the list goes on and on.

How Lyme disease relates to Morgellons Disease

I noted the connection with Lyme disease when I first became aware of MD in 2003. As reported earlier in this book, 97% of my MD study group had been diagnosed with Lyme disease, either through positive blood work or high clinical suspicion. In addition to the various skin symptoms described in an earlier chapter, almost all MD patients have symptoms that are classic for Lyme disease including extreme fatigue, malaise, mental confusion, insomnia, muscle and joint pain, muscle twitches, and neuropathies.

Fibroblasts are cells that produce collagen and, as discussed earlier, it has been proposed that fibroblasts are where the proliferation of collagen, seen in Morgellons disease, begins. As long ago as 1992, Georgilis, Peakcocke & Klempner reported that fibroblasts protect *Bb* from antibiotics and provide a place where the spirochetes can continue to survive. In 1993, Klempner, Noring & Rogers reported the ability of

Bb to adhere to, penetrate and invade human fibroblasts. The fact that *Borrelia* bacteria have an affinity for collagen has been demonstrated in several papers, including one by Wood et al in 2015 (see bibliography).

Further strengthening the Lyme association, the work of Middelveen et al showed positive tests for *Bb* in 24 of 25 MD patients sampled and the work of Dr. Jyotsna Shah of IGeneX found either *Bb* or another related *Borrelia* in all of the 10 subjects in her pilot study. Dr. Eva Sapi found *Bb* to be one of 2 pathogens that she consistently found in her MD subjects even in the metagenomic sequencing she had performed at PerkinElmer Biotechnology Company in Waltham, Massachusetts.

Many people mistakenly believe that Lyme disease is a relatively new phenomenon. Although the name "Lyme disease" and the fact that it is caused by *Borrelia burgdorferi* came to attention in the late 20th century, human infection by the *Bb* spirochete has been around for thousands of years as evidenced by the fact that *Bb* was found in the knees of "Otzi the ice man", the 5000 year old mummy found frozen in a northern Italian glacier in 1991. There may not have been a catchy name for the disease until 1975 and an awareness of the causative pathogen until 1982 but even people incorrectly diagnosed with DOP in the early 1900s could have been infected with the *Bb* spirochete that causes what we now know as Lyme disease.

It is tempting to assume that Morgellons disease is a dermatological manifestation of Lyme disease based on what we know so far. The association is certainly there. But there is still the possibility that MD may be discovered to be yet another in a growing list of co-infections of Lyme disease, spread by ticks and possibly other biting vectors. Not to disprove the assertion that MD is a manifestation of Lyme, but in an attempt to look at the situation objectively, I will review some of the findings that may lend doubt to the Lyme causation theory of MD.

Playing Devil's Advocate to the Lyme Causation Theory

The presence of a bacterium in an ill patient does not *necessarily* mean that the bacterium is the cause of the patient's symptoms. This was dramatically demonstrated more than 20 years ago when it was surmised that Epstein-Barr Virus (EBV) was the cause of Chronic Fatigue Syndrome (CFS). Because EBV titers were elevated in CFS patients, patients were told that EBV *caused* their illness. Years later we learned that EBV titers are present in nearly everyone and rise opportunistically when the immune system is challenged. **Correlation does not imply causation.**

After a cursory look at the search engine PubMed, I was able to find journal articles reporting 10 other skin conditions in which biopsies of lesions were culture positive for *B.*

burgdorferi spirochetes when the patient also happened to have Lyme disease. *B. burgdorferi* were found in the skin biopsies of patients with the following skin conditions when the same patients were seropositive for Bb (Lyme):

Cutaneous sarcoidosis

Prurigo Pigmentosa

Granuloma Annulare

Necrobiosis lipoidica

Necrobiotic xanthogranuloma

Erythema annulare centrifugum

Interstitial granulomatous dermatitis

Mycosis fungoides

Lobular panniculitis

Cutaneous scleroderma

Some may claim that this indicates that all of the above-named dermatoses are *caused* by the spirochete that causes Lyme disease, in other words, that they are dermatological manifestations of Lyme. This seems unlikely to me. A more likely explanation, based upon our awareness that *Bb* spirochetes tend to seek out weakened and injured parts of the body, is that the *Bb* that caused these patients' systemic Lyme disease was drawn to their co-existing dermatoses. Is this the same case with *Bb* in Morgellons lesions? We are not yet prepared to answer this question definitively.

Later, in the chapter on treatment, I will explain that Lyme disease treatment does not cure MD patients. Treatment that focuses on management of the bacterial infection *Bartonellosis* has a much higher clinical efficacy. Eight *Bartonella* species and subspecies are known to cause disease in humans. *Bartonellosis* can be transmitted by cat scratches or by the bites of ticks, mosquitos, sand flies or fleas. (Interestingly, many Morgellons patients recount that their symptoms began following a flea infestation.) *Bartonella henselae* was the most frequently found of 4 pathogens identified in MD lesions by Dr. Randy Wymore. Besides *Borrelia*, Dr. Shah of IGeneX found *Bartonella* in 3 out of 10 subjects in her pilot study. Please note that I am not suggesting that *Bartonella* bacteria **cause** Morgellons disease. I am just noting that there are other bacteria besides Bb that are associated with it.

Furthermore, if Lyme disease causes MD, why do only 6% of Lyme patients become ill with MD symptoms? This could be due to immune susceptibilities or genetic predispositions but it still leaves pause to wonder.

I am not claiming to know what causes Morgellons disease nor am I in a position to positively refute another's premise. However, I feel it important to keep an open mind and not be trapped by logical fallacies as has often happened in medical research. I am the first person who brought the correlation of Morgellons disease and Lyme disease to public attention; however, I still do not think that we can say with certainty what this correlation implies.

Part Five

Swimming Against the Tide

*"Do what you feel in your heart to be right-
for you'll be criticized anyway. You'll be
damned if you do, and damned if you don't."*

— **Eleanor Roosevelt**

TRIALS AND TRIBULATIONS
OF A TROUBLE MAKER

"First, they ignore you, then they laugh at you, then they fight you, then you win". (One of the 10 most famous quotes that no one ever said).

Philosopher Thomas Kuhn proposed that scientific communities operate within a rigid set of assumptions and therefore are not susceptible to a paradigm shift when confronted by an anomaly. Since the beginning of time, anyone with a radically new idea in the field of science or medicine (or in any field, for that matter) has been ridiculed and persecuted. It comes with the territory.

During the early years of my involvement with MD, when none of my colleagues believed or showed interest in what I was seeing in these unusual patients, I experienced times of disillusionment, especially when I heard derogatory comments about me. In his book *Chaos: Making a New Science,* James Gleick writes:

"Ideas that require people to reorganize their picture of the world provoke hostility." Provoke I did. And hostility surely followed.

I was raising my children at the time and they were upset when they would read negative things about me on the Internet. I was being called a quack and was said to be taking advantage of patients or even killing patients with my treatment methods. My children knew that nothing could be further from the truth. But they worried, as did Bill Pitt, that I might meet some kind of terrible fate for sticking to my guns and refusing to accept what I knew to be wrong. I regret that my children had to endure those difficult times but now that they are adults they admit that seeing their mother stand up for what she believed to be right was a lesson of value that far outweighed any discomfort they may have experienced.

Added to these frustrations was the daunting fact that I was treating a disease with no known cause and no accepted treatment. Despite the impediments, I could not in good conscience let these patients suffer without trying something, anything to help. Patients signed treatment consent forms indicating that they were fully aware of the experimental nature of the treatment. These were desperate people and desperate times call for desperate measures. Every single one of my MD patients told me that they would gladly try any treatment, even if it posed a 50% risk of death. They were at a point where all they wanted to do was get better or die.

Of course, all of my treatments were with FDA-approved medications and I never tried anything that I thought would pose a danger. I followed patients' lab work monthly and was available to them around the clock to answer their emails about any side effects or problems with the medications. My actions were seen as reckless only because I was not following the standard of care in terms of what is known as evidenced based medicine (more about this in a following chapter). The medications I was prescribing were not "indicated" for MD. But how could they have been? The disease didn't "exist"!

Actually, rather than harming patients, I was saving many patients from the disastrous consequences of self-medicating with caustic, toxic chemicals. Morgellons patients were doing things like ingesting turpentine and mothballs, dousing their skin in gasoline or lawn fertilizer and putting lighter fluid on their lesions and lighting them on fire. These actions were driven by an intense desire for relief but, not surprisingly, were interpreted by the medical community as more indications of mental instability.

Furthermore, I was helping patients by taking care of their basic care needs. Many would no longer see their PCP for check-ups or any other reason because they did not want to be lectured about their skin and accused of self-mutilation. Female MD patients have told me that they have not had pap smears or mammograms for 10 years or more because of their embarrassing and painful lesions and their desire not to be questioned about them.

Treating a "nonexistent" disease with antimicrobials was not highly looked upon by the regulatory boards and health insurance companies balked at the unheard of combinations of medications I was prescribing for off-label use. Sometimes health insurers refused to pay, leaving patients to suffer, but as long as I saw that a medication was helping I kept pushing to have it covered. Unfortunately, some patients had no insurance or had a large deductible to meet, obligating me to use a medication combination that did not work as well. To add to these obstructions, struggling to defend my treatment decisions in order to maintain my professional license consumed my time, energy and finances and was not something that my training had prepared me to do.

Even the dermatologists who thought MD might indeed be a physiological condition warned me that it was unethical to treat a condition without knowledge of the cause. I would answer, "Then what do you propose we do with these patients?" I was told to do nothing until a cause or cure could be discovered. In my opinion, it was unethical to leave these patients to suffer for who-knows-how-many years without trying to help. But I must admit that it was nerve wracking not having a protocol to follow or an expert to consult.

There were days when I wanted to give up. I was beaten down with the criticisms and overwhelmed with the huge responsibility of taking care of these very ill patients without support. It's tiring to swim against the tide. For moral support, I taped the following Dr. Martin Luther King quote to my desk and read it several times during the day when I was in my office. It became my guiding mantra.

"Cowardice asks the question - is it safe?
Expediency asks the question - is it politic?
Vanity asks the question - is it popular?
But conscience asks the question - is it right?
And there comes a time when one must take a
position That is neither safe, nor politic, nor popular
But one must take it because it is right."

— Dr. Martin Luther King

PSEUDOSCIENCE VERSUS SCIENCE: WHERE DO WE DRAW THE LINE?

Hypotheses are proposed explanations for natural phenomena. The scientific method is a process that includes formulating a logical and testable hypothesis, controlling for confounding variables and experimenter bias as much as possible, and executing unbiased testing, the results of which support or do not support the hypothesis. (Note that experimental results are not said to **prove** or **disprove** a hypothesis).

Pseudoscience, on the other hand, is described as a collection of conjectures or theories that cannot be accepted or refuted using the scientific method. This sounds pretty clear-cut but, in reality, there is a fuzzy line between science and pseudoscience. No matter how deeply based in logic a hypothesis may be or how many repeated observations it is based upon, it is not always possible to test it due to ethical or logistical impediments. If testing cannot be performed, does this mean that a theory is based on pseudoscience?

Not necessarily. The ultimate discerning feature between science and pseudoscience, as proposed by Karl Popper, a 20th-century philosopher of science, is whether a hypothesis passes the test for *falsifiability*. This discerning criterion is still widely used by scientists today. Falsifiability means that it is possible to conceive of an argument that could refute the proposed hypothesis. For example, if a hypothesis states that all swans are white, the discovery of even one black swan would immediately refute the hypothesis, meaning that the hypothesis passes the test for falsifiability and cannot be considered pseudoscience.

It is believed that pseudoscientists promote unfalsifiable theories that they declare to be scientifically true. An example of a pseudoscience theory would be: "Morgellons disease has been sent down to us from aliens in outer space to slowly wipe out our planet". This hypothesis cannot be supported or refuted. However, the hypothesis that Morgellons disease is caused by the Lyme bacteria *Bb* is **not** pseudoscience. It is an idea that can be tested and supported or refuted. Researchers have already taken the first step in testing this hypothesis by showing the presence of *Bb* in the lesions of MD patients. As research continues, the next step will be a systematic process to support or refute *Bb* as the **cause** of MD.

However, even the test for falsifiability does not always make a clear demarcation between science and pseudoscience. There are many elegant and widely accepted theories that have not and cannot pass the test of falsifiability. One example is string theory, a theory that has been accepted and respected by theoretical physicists. String theory, in the strictest definition, should be considered pseudoscience since there is no way to refute the theory using the scientific method. But in the case of string theory, the fact that it is logical, intellectually supported, and widely accepted by experts in the field leads to it not being seen as pseudoscience.

Quantum theory is a respected theory in the field of physics. However, when the ideas of quantum thinking are transposed into medicine (energy healing, for example) the medical elite routinely labels these ideas as pseudoscience rather than showing intellectual curiosity about a possible new paradigm of medicine. I have trouble understanding quantum theory and how it relates to medicine myself but I do not refute it out of hand. I find it more appropriate to say, "I don't understand it".

As a person who has always been open to new ideas, I take issue with the medical community hastily labeling new ways of thinking about health as pseudoscience. Many of the new approaches to health care being used by holistic or integrated doctors are valuable additions to the arsenal of techniques used to diagnose and treat disease. These new approaches are often based upon nothing more than repeated clinical observations and have therefore not been studied using the scientific method. However, repeated clinical observations are not completely without merit in the world of scientific inquiry and may, in fact, form the basis of new testable hypotheses. Just because a theory has not run the gauntlet of the scientific method does not *necessarily* make it pseudoscience.

Michael D. Gordon, Ph.D., professor of scientific history at Princeton, writes in his book *The Pseudoscience Wars* that "individual scientists (as distinct from the monolithic 'scientific community') designate a doctrine a 'pseudoscience' only when they perceive themselves to be threatened—not necessarily by the new ideas themselves, but by what those ideas represent about the authority of science, science's access to resource or some other broader social trend. If one is not threatened, there is no need to lash out at the perceived pseudoscience; instead, one continues with one's work and happily ignores the cranks."

Pseudoscience clearly incites an angry and appalled reaction whereas poorly executed science is simply discounted. Conservative thinkers who do not like their worldview challenged incite the backlash to new ideas that threaten the status quo. Those of us who are interested in new information that challenges current thought are considered to be "on the fringe". We prefer to think of ourselves as being "on the cutting edge"!

The bastion of medical conservancy considers the concept of Morgellons disease to be pseudoscience or "fringe medicine" not only because its existence is based on the observations of a few renegade clinicians and researchers but clearly because it seems implausible and illogical within medicine's current framework of understanding.

In summary, there is a fine line between what is considered science and pseudoscience. In a textbook sense, a theory may be called pseudoscience if its premise is not testable. However, the scientific community accepts some untestable theories. A criterion for defining pseudoscience has never been that a premise is strange, hard-to-believe, or unlikely.

So, it appears to come down to this: in practice, an idea is being considered pseudoscience when:

1. Its premise seems highly unlikely by the medical establishment and
2. The top scientists in the idea's particular field do not subscribe to it.

To assure that Morgellons disease is not viewed as pseudoscience but rather as a respected scientific model of disease it appears that what is needed is:

1. An elegant and logical sounding theory of etiology and pathological mechanisms, that has been tested using the scientific method, and

2. Prominent thinkers in the field of medicine, particularly in the areas of dermatology and psychiatry, embracing and supporting the theory.

With meager funds at their disposal, a few devoted researchers are working towards #1. This book along with continued awareness campaigns by the CEHMDF and a documentary-in-the-making by Pi Ware (morgellonsmovie.org) are aiming towards #2.

In the next chapter, we will discuss skepticism and how it relates to the scientific method. We will see that skepticism, by definition, involves using the scientific method to determine the truth or significance of a claim. Neither science nor skepticism should involve prejudice or bias of the observer. These are emotions, and there is no room for emotion in science.

REFUTING THE SKEPTICS

We have come to think of a skeptic as a negative person who will not believe anything unless it is obvious or concrete. Actually, skepticism is defined by Brian Dunning of *The Skeptoid* as *"the process of finding a supported conclusion, not the justification of a preconceived conclusion"*.

The skeptics of Morgellons as a legitimate disease have not gone through the process of looking into the research in order to support or refute it. What they have exhibited is a knee-jerk reaction to something that sounds implausible. Skepticism should not be about debunking – it should be a rational and thoughtful process that aims for the truth based on testable findings.

Since skeptics, in the purest sense of the term, arrive at conclusions through the scientific method, they do not see anecdotal information or personal accounts as valuable to their process. So, the answers I list below to the doubts I often hear are not going to change the mind of a true skeptic. What I hope to do is **open** their minds, so that they may take the time to investigate rather than simply to discredit.

The skeptics say...

"These patients are delusional! Don't waste your time with them!"

However...

I have examined children as young as 9 months old with objective signs of Morgellons disease. There are no documented cases of delusional 9-month-old babies! In a previous chapter, I have described in detail the differences between delusions of parasitosis and MD.

The skeptics say…

"These lesions are caused by aggressive scratching and picking."

However…

The lesions are often seen in places on the back where patients cannot reach to scratch. Furthermore, I have spoken with a gastroenterologist in Boston who has found unusual lesions in the colons of 2 different MD patients. He told me that the lesions he saw in these patients' colons were like nothing he has ever seen before on colonoscopy. The California gynecologist of another of my MD patients was amazed to see unusual lesions in the patient's uterus saying that she had never seen anything similar in her 20-year career.

The skeptics say…

"Those filaments are nothing more than textile threads that are stuck to the lesions!"

However…

In 2006, forensic scientist Ron Pogue at the Tulsa Police Crime Lab in Oklahoma checked a Morgellons filament sample against known substances in the Federal Bureau of Investigation (FBI) national database. The lab's director, Mark Boese, said that the filaments were "consistent with something that the body may be producing." He added, "These filaments cannot be manmade and do not come from a plant. This could be a byproduct of a biological organism.". In fact, recent research by Middelveen et al has found the filaments to be composed of the body's own proteins collagen and keratin, as described in an earlier chapter.

The skeptics say…

"The filaments are shoved under the skin by the patient."

However…

It would be physically impossible for anyone to implant filaments under their skin as deeply rooted and difficult to extract as these filaments are. Furthermore, the filaments are found under the skin in places that a patient cannot even reach. (One dermatologist's answer to this was that the patient's spouse must have been inserting the filaments!). Moreover, I have spoken with a gynecologist in Chicago who has reported removing filaments from the cervixes of 2 women with MD and an ophthalmologist in San Francisco has removed filaments from the eyes of one of my MD patients. Another of my MD patients had a lymph node removed and the pathology report stated there was a red "thread" in the lymph gland.

In summary, there is too much clinical and scientific evidence for anyone to continue doubting Morgellons as a physiological disease. It is time for skeptics to cast aside their unsubstantiated doubts and pay attention to what they see and hear.

*"In the face of obvious physical
abnormalities, skepticism is inappropriate"*
(Richard Shoemaker, M.D.)

"EVIDENCED BASED MEDICINE": WHERE IS THE EVIDENCE FOR IT?

The current use of the term "evidence based medicine" means that a treatment has been tested in randomized, controlled trials, using equally matched, double-blinded, placebo-controlled study groups. Evidence-based practice (EBP) is defined by the Institute of Medicine (2001) as the integration of 1. Best-researched evidence, 2. Clinical expertise, and 3. Patient values. Thus, EBP would be in contrast to a medical practice based on tradition, convention, belief, or anecdotal evidence. EBP has become the gold standard to which most medical practices aspire.

There are those in health care who believe that the medical field has become overly invested in the idea that all procedures and treatments should be evidence based in order to be considered legitimate for clinical use. The importance of the 2nd and 3rd aspects of EBP –

clinical expertise and patient values – is being overlooked.

There is no doubt that evidence that is based on randomized, double-blinded, placebo-controlled studies is an application of the scientific method at its finest. However, this rigorous testing is often not feasible. For one thing, it is sometimes unethical (for example, putting very ill patients in a control group thereby denying them a possible cure). In other incidences, there are simply too many confounding variables to result in a meaningful outcome.

There are many regularly used medications and treatment options that are not evidence based in the sense described above. Acetylsalicylic acid (ASA), commonly known as Aspirin (a *Bayer* trademark), is an over-the-counter pain relief medication that is one of the most commonly used medications in the world. Often recommended by physicians, ASA has been in use for thousands of years and it is used because it has always worked, not because it has been tested according to the principles of evidence-based-medicine. If a treatment is effective, widely used and appears to do no harm isn't this evidence enough of its clinical worth?

Eminence Based Medicine

In reality, what is known as "eminence based medicine" often trumps evidenced based medicine in the world of day-to-day medical practice. Eminence based medicine relies on the clinical expertise of respected specialists or those who have been in practice for many years. In his August 2, 2016 "CardioBrief" column in the online magazine, *MEDPAGE Today,* Larry Husten writes:

"…..the responsibility for eminence-based medicine goes well beyond the elite coterie of experts. The real problem is the culture of medicine, which rewards the hubris of eminence and actively punishes or offers subtle disincentives to anyone who questions this process. … Medical training is disturbingly similar to military training, where immediate and

unreflecting obedience is the goal. …… In both, the submission to authority is a central tenet."

Eminence Based Medicine in Action

When PPIs (proton pump inhibitors) first came on the market in the late 1980s they were indicated to inhibit gastric acid secretion for the purpose of healing severe gastrointestinal reflux and stomach ulcers. This means that the clinical trials for PPIs showed efficacy and safety for short-term (approximate 2 week) use of the medication. However, throughout the past 25 years, gastroenterologists have increasingly prescribed PPIs for long-term or permanent use by patients with heartburn. This use of PPIs is off-label since the drug was not indicated to *permanently* inhibit stomach acid production. Since obstruction of acid production is a convenient and quick fix for patients with heartburn, long-term use of PPIs has become almost standard of care. In fact, it has filtered down from the "expertise" of gastroenterologists to the day-to-day practice of primary care, despite the fact that the use of PPIs on a permanent basis is not evidenced-based and probably even dangerous.

Acid is needed for proper digestion and shutting down acid production for the relatively brief time it takes to heal an ulcer makes sense. Turning acid production off permanently does not. Because PPIs were never tested for long-term use, we do not know how severely malnourished this patient group may have become. Furthermore, a search of PubMed.com reveals numerous peer-reviewed articles regarding the relationship between long-term use of PPIs and stomach cancer. This example of the current clinical use of PPIs demonstrates that evidenced based medicine is extolled when politic and yet overlooked by experts when clinically convenient to do so.

Interestingly, alternative practitioners of what the medical establishment calls "fringe" medicine have discovered that about a third of people with heartburn actually have an acid

deficit rather than an acid surplus, a condition known as hypochlorhydria. Patients with hypochlorhydria have heartburn because their food sits undigested in the stomach for too long since the stomach does not contain enough acid to propel the food along the digestive tract. When these patients take hydrochloric acid tablets with their meals, their heartburn disappears. The double blind, placebo-controlled trials are not there – but giving a patient hydrochloric acid is both a diagnosis and a treatment. If it helps, the patient has hypochlorhydria. Physicians scoff at practitioners who suggest that hypochlorhydria is a rampant problem but no one is watch-guarding the gastroenterologists who abuse PPIs. This is an example of eminence based medicine, defined in the tongue-in-cheek, *A Skeptic's Medical Dictionary*, as "making the same mistakes with increasing confidence over an impressive number of years."

In short, the medical establishment derides those who practice medicine that is not evidence based and considers it malpractice to prescribe treatments in a different way or for a different purpose than their FDA designated indication. Clearly, however, this does not reflect what actually goes on in clinical practice. My point is that condemning those of us who treat Morgellons patients with off-label use of antibiotics is hypocritical when off-label use of treatments takes place in doctors' offices every day. We may not be fulfilling the "best-researched evidence" part of the criteria for evidenced-based-practice, but those of us who regularly work with MD patients are fulfilling the criteria of clinical expertise and patient values.

Medical decision-making should be left to the discretion of individual health care providers enabling them to make the best decisions for their patients based on patient needs, situation and response. This is what they have been trained to do. If health care decisions were nothing more than algorithms, we would be able to go to a Robot for our health care. Likewise, patients should be allowed to choose among treatment options based upon informed consent.

As medical decision-making is increasingly being taken over by insurance companies it has become ever more exasperating to practice medicine. But the ultimate travesty lies in what is happening to the patients. When their health care providers' hands are tied to provide them with the best care for their unique case, patients suffer and sometimes die.

Dr. Benjamin Rush, a signer of the Declaration of Independence and personal physician to President George Washington, predicted this medical crisis. In his introductory remarks to a course lecture at the University of Pennsylvania on November 3, 1801, he listed 24 "causes, which have retarded the progress of our science". The 22nd cause read:

"Conferring exclusive privileges upon bodies of physicians, and forbidding men of equal talents and knowledge, under severe penalties from practicing

medicine within certain districts of cities and countries. Such institutions, however sanctioned by ancient charters and names, are the bastiles of our science."

It is unfortunate that Dr. Rush's brilliant foresight about the dangers inherent in medical elitism did not prompt him to insist on a provision in the Declaration of Independence to protect patients' "right to choose."

Part Six

Frequently Asked Questions

"The important thing is to not stop questioning."

— Albert Einstein

IS MORGELLONS DISEASE CONTAGIOUS?

Whether person-to-person transmission is a concern with Morgellons disease is a question that has raised tremendous anxiety in both patients and health care workers. Most patients report no symptoms in their loved ones despite the fact that they continue to sleep with their spouses and care for their children throughout their illnesses. Sadly, many patients with symptoms of MD have become hermits, afraid of contaminating their environment or spreading their disease to friends, family, and even total strangers. I once took care of an MD patient who had not hugged her own son for 5 years due to her fear of contaminating him.

Eighteen percent of my MD patients have reported at least one family member with symptoms similar to theirs. Patients often ask, "If it is not contagious, why do several people in my family have it?" I believe strongly that this is due to common exposure to the source of contagion.

Most of the patients with close family members who share their symptoms report that symptoms started after one of the following situations affecting all family members: a lice or flea infestation in the home; common exposure to dirty water; recent return from a 3rd world country, or camping. It bears noting that I did not examine subjects' family members reported as having symptoms and so they may not have actually had Morgellons disease. I have noticed a tendency for MD patients to fear and suspect that family members are also infected, despite their denial of symptoms.

Patients say "I know this is contagious because when I'm in a group of people I notice everyone close to me begins scratching their nose, eyes, face or head." Please know that the filaments themselves are not contaminants – think of them as "debris" or byproducts of the infection but they are not infectious agents. However, filaments are sometimes expelled into the air from an MD victim and become irritants to those around them. This is why MD patients notice people around them scratching – the filaments are irritating to mucous membranes and delicate skin. Whenever I see an MD patient in my office I notice that my staff and I feel itchy for 15 to 20 minutes after the patient leaves. However, this sensation subsides as the filaments in the air begin to settle down.

In summary, here is what we know so far about contagiousness: Morgellons disease is not spread through casual human contact. Sufferers do not need to worry about infecting people who ride the bus with them or friends who accompany them to dinner. Whatever the causative pathogen may be, it needs to get underneath the skin to contaminate the victim. Symptoms begin after a bite or other type of puncture wound or introduction of contaminated water or dirt into an opening on the skin such as a non-healed cut or open lesion. Is it sexually transmitted? We do not yet know the definitive answer to this question but many patients with severe disease have continued to have sexual relations with their partner while the partner remains asymptomatic.

If Morgellons disease were spread by casual contact, I would surely have contracted it by now. I have examined close to a thousand MD patients since 2003, without using any special precautions, and I have not developed the symptoms, even though I have a personal history of Lyme disease.

One of my most difficult tasks is convincing MD patients that people around them are not at risk of contracting their disease. This is very important for patients to know because human contact is crucial for psychological and physical wellbeing. Morgellons patients should reach out to others for help and comfort and family and friends should not be afraid to hug and support their loved ones with MD.

SHOULD PATIENTS DISINFECT THEIR HOMES?

Quite a few MD patients report that they spend many hours a day on decontamination routines, cleaning and disinfecting their homes. They vacuum several times per day, change the sheets on their beds daily, wash clothes with scalding hot water and tirelessly scrub and clean. Their personal hygiene routines are exhaustive too. Patients have told me that they spend 2 to 3 hours at night performing self-care rituals just to get ready for bed. Many MD patients are convinced that pests in their environment are causing their symptoms and believe that eliminating them is the only way to get well. I have had patients who are financially able to do so move from place to place to "escape" their torturers.

The CEHMDF nurses and I advise patients against doing this. These cleaning rituals do **not** help and they never have. Furthermore, these routines are exhausting, taking away precious energy and creating stress for a person who is trying to heal. Remember that the fibers and other exudates are **not** infective agents and will not re-infect a patient or contaminate anyone else. **The cause of MD patients' torment is within them, not around them.**

ARE PETS VULNERABLE?

Many people have reported that their pets have lesions and filaments consistent with MD. So far we have heard reports of cats, dogs and horses with the characteristic lesions and filaments. Since animals are not known to be delusional, this finding should serve as more evidence that MD is not a delusional disorder. People often wonder what they should do for their pets with this disease. The first step would be to visit a

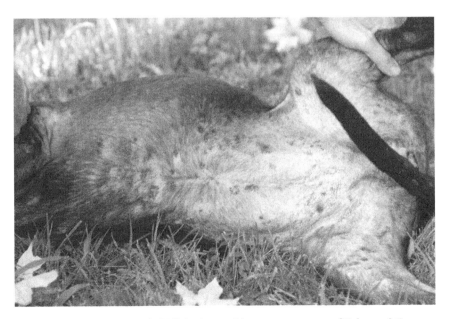

Image 45: Dog with MD lesions. Photo courtesy of Edward C. Rasmussen

veterinarian and provide him/her with information about Morgellons disease. Ask that your pet be tested for Lyme disease. Lyme disease is very rare in cats (although they are vulnerable to other tickborne diseases) but common enough in horses and dogs. If your pet is positive for Lyme disease the vet will treat with antibiotics and hopefully the antibiotics will help the MD.

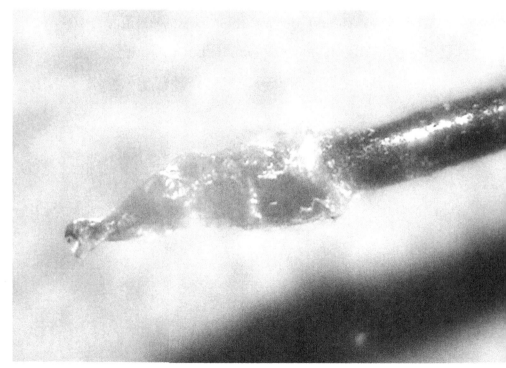

Image 46: Dog whisker with gelatinous material at the root, similar to what is seen in humans with MD. Photo courtesy of Lee M. Laskowsky

WHY ARE SOME PATIENTS SICKER THAN OTHERS?

There is a huge range in presentation of MD patients from those with no lesions and minor symptoms all the way to those who are completely disfigured and disabled by their disease. No one knows for sure why this is the case. In all disease states, a weak immune status in the host facilitates more serious disease. I assume that this is the case with MD as well. Furthermore, genetic research continues to reveal new information about genetic predispositions to different types of maladies. In fact, we may even discover that the causative pathogen of Morgellons disease is ubiquitous with only a small segment of the (immune-suppressed and/or genetically susceptible) population vulnerable to its effects.

The worst case I ever saw of MD was a man who needed to take high daily doses of prednisone in order to manage his autoimmune disease. Prednisone is an immune suppressant and when taken over a long period of time allows infections of many kinds to go unchecked. This patient had lesions that were 3 to 4 inches in diameter and his response to treatment was minimal. He eventually succumbed to his autoimmune disease. I have treated other MD patients who were on immune suppressant medications or had AIDS (acquired immune deficiency syndrome). These patients are particularly resistant to treatment. This is why an important aspect of treatment is doing everything possible to strengthen and relieve burdens from the immune system.

DO ALL MORGELLONS DISEASE PATIENTS HAVE LESIONS?

As mentioned in the last chapter, MD is highly variable in presentation with the one constant being the presence of sub-dermal filaments. I have examined many MD patients who have symptoms of biting, stinging, crawling and itching and have filaments under the skin seen with careful examination but who do NOT have visible lesions. In a sense, these are the lucky ones because they do not have to worry about the reaction of people who see them in public. I would guestimate that about 15 - 20% of my Morgellons patients do not have lesions. And others have only a few. The reason for this is unknown but is most likely a factor of the previously discussed topic – certain people are just more affected by the disease than others.

So, in a word, the answer to the question posed in the title is "no". Not all Morgellons disease patients have lesions. Again, the filaments are the deciding factor in a Morgellons disease diagnosis. Unfortunately, some patients who actually have MD may not even know they have filaments if they have not carefully examined their skin with lighted magnification.

IS MORGELLONS DISEASE FATAL?

Since I have been treating Morgellons disease, 10 of my patients have died but they have not succumbed to the physical illness itself. Most commonly, patients have accidentally taken too many sedating medications in search of relief of their pain, insomnia, and heightened anxiety. In two cases I am sure that the patients overdosed due to severe cognitive dysfunction and likely forgot that they had already taken their sleeping pills and took them again. An 88-year-old MD patient of mine died of a heart attack and two patients died due to the illness that caused them to have to take immune suppressants (autoimmune disease and organ transplant). One died of colon cancer. There are a couple of cases where I suspected suicide.

I cannot say for certain that MD is never fatal but it would appear that way from what I have seen so far. This would support the notion that the cause is parasitic in nature. As was discussed earlier, bacteria, nematodes, arthropods, worms and fungi can all be parasites but parasitic bacteria are the parasites suspected in the causation of MD. A parasite does not define the type of pathogen but merely that the pathogen cannot live without the host. It would be counterproductive for a parasite to intentionally kill its host.

Part Seven

Healing the Wounded

"There are many medicines and cures for all kinds of sick people. But, unless kind hands are given in service and generous hearts are given in love, I do not think there can ever be a cure for the terrible sickness of feeling unloved."

— Mother Teresa

THERE IS HOPE

Pending more understanding of the cause and risk factors, a total cure for Morgellons disease is elusive. Treatment focuses on symptom management and, when a patient is willing (and most are), treatment with experimental combinations of antibiotics, antifungals, antiparasitics, and anthelminthics. Many have improved with treatment but not without enduring temporary symptom intensification and the need for frequent medication changes due to an apparently uncanny ability of the organism to adapt or mutate. Every patient is unique so treatment involves trial and error and months of frustration for both the patient and the practitioner.

In patients who have had symptoms for less than a year or whose symptoms are not severe, I see a vast improvement after about a year of treatment. Treatment of serious or long-lasting cases has taken as long as 6 years. Most patients' recoveries happen somewhere in between the two extremes with an average of 2-3 years.

All of the MD patients I have treated have improved – the difference is in the amount of improvement and the time it takes to get there. About 5 to 10% of my patients have become completely asymptomatic after treatment and have stayed that way for as long as 5 years. The majority of my treated patients are left with some residual symptoms but their situation is vastly improved and they are able to function and live a normal life. About 10-15% improve very little. These tend to be the patients with the most serious symptoms who have been sick a very long time or have environmental or psychosocial stresses suppressing their immune systems.

So, there is definitely hope, and this point should be stressed to every patient with this disease. Patients have a higher chance of recovery when they are strictly compliant with the treatment protocol and do everything they can to strengthen their immune systems (more about this in the chapter on treatment). The difficult part is sticking with the long treatment. It takes a real leap of faith. But those who have beaten the disease say that this is what is needed: faith and a stubborn refusal to give in.

SYMPTOM MANAGEMENT

This chapter focuses solely on symptom management rather than treatment methods. The symptoms of MD are so stressful for the patient that relieving them becomes an important part of the overall treatment. Reduction of discomfort and anxiety allows the immune system to function more effectively.

These are products that have been successfully used by my patients over the years. I have no financial interest in any of the products for which name brands are given. OTC indicates "over-the-counter" and Rx means that a prescription is needed. All of these suggestions are based upon feedback from my patients; I cannot personally endorse them but can report that they have been helpful to others.

1. Soaps and other body cleansers

    a. Sulfur soap (found in stores with Mexican products – also in many Walmarts), (OTC)

    b. Hexachlorophene 3% liquid cleanser, (Rx)

2. Topical disinfectants to put on lesions

    a. Everclear (95-100% grain alcohol – found in liquor stores but illegal in some states) – use topically!

    b. Betadine (OTC)

    c. Gentian violet (OTC)

    d. Merthiolate tincture (OTC)

3. Head

    a. Selsun Blue shampoo – wash scalp AND body with this. There is an OTC version and a stronger Rx one

    b. Nioxin Scalp Recovery Medicating Cleanser (shampoo) and conditioner (OTC)

c. Add a few drops of Oregano oil to shampoo and/or rub some into the scalp to relieve itchiness (OTC)

d. Horse shampoo available at animal feed stores (OTC)

e. Garlic shampoo and garlic conditioner from the Vermont Country Store www.vermontcountrystore.com (no bad smell!) (OTC)

4. Mouth

a. Biotene mouthwash (OTC)

b. Tea tree oil mouthwash (OTC)

c. Grapefruit seed extract tincture mixed with a few ounces of water – swish and swallow

d. Coconut oil, swished in mouth for 20 minutes

e. Important to see a dentist every 3 months for teeth cleaning

5. Topical antibiotic creams, ointments, etc (All work for only a few weeks)

    a. Gentamycin ointment (Rx)

    b. Silvadene (Rx cream with silver and sulfa)

    c. Anti-fungal creams, like Lotrimin (OTC)

    d. Sulfur cream (OTC). (Walmart or Mexican stores)

6. Soaks

    a. Mineral salts – 1 c in hot bath water (OTC)

    b. Vick's Vapo Steam Liquid – use the entire bottle in hot water bath (OTC)

    c. LL Magnetic Clay in hot water bath. www.magneticclay.com or diatomaceous earth or zeolite (OTC)

7. Topicals to "bring things out"

    a. Tea Tree Oil (OTC).

    b. Ichthammol ointment (drawing salve) OTC but ask your pharmacist

c. Preparation H (OTC)

d. Homeopathic Rescue Cream (OTC)

e. Wart medicine containing salicylic acid (OTC)

f. Redmond Real Salt Clay Powder from vitacost.com. Mix with water to make a poultice (or just buy a chunk of Redmond Rock and rub it on the skin. This is OTC and can be found at feed stores or online.)

8. Soothing topicals

a. Neosporin Pain Relief cream or ointment (OTC)

b. DermaZinc Cream (OTC)

c. Vick's Vapo Rub (OTC)

d. Biafine topical emulsion (Rx)

e. Pure shea butter (OTC)

9. To heal lesions quickly

a. Dercut ("dare-KOOT") ointment (OTC, order online)

b. HY-TAPE – a pink, zinc-oxide-impregnated tape that helps the wounds heal faster, feel better and not form the hard scabs. OTC/ Info here: www.hytape.com

c. Cordran tape (Rx) – apply to lesions every 12 hours

d. Kenalog intra-lesion injections – must be done in a doctor's office

10. To remove tough, calloused skin and hard scabs (debride)

a. Santyl ointment (collagenase), (Rx)

b. Nature's Gift Debriding Soap (OTC – find online)

c. Redmond Rock rubbed back and forth over the hard skin (OTC)

11. Anti-itch medications

a. Zonalon cream (Rx topical Doxepin – can be sedating)

b. Eurax cream (Rx) for itchy skin and for scabies

c. 999 Itch Relief Skin Ointment (OTC) (available in Asian stores)

d. OTC antihistamines

b. Doxepin tablets, sedating, take at night (Rx)

12. To fade scarring and discolorations
Dermal K Cream by Dixie Health, OTC, order online

13. Diet and Supplements

a. Cut out sugars and white flour

b. Garlic supplements or, better yet, whole raw garlic cloves every day

c. Ginger tincture

d. Gotu Kola and Grape Seed extract – both good for healing skin

b. Biotin (OTC) – vitamin particularly good for the skin

14. Procedures – ask your dermatologist about these. (Some will not be possible while there are active lesions)

    a. Cold laser therapies

    b. Intense pulse light (offered in many spas specializing in skin treatments). This will help remove the scars after treatment

    c. Blue Light Therapy (Blu-U, Clear Light)

    d. Far infrared halogen heaters for at-home sauna treatments

TREATMENT

First and foremost, health care providers have the power to alleviate the suffering of MD patients by simply validating the reality of their symptoms, responding to them with empathy, and expressing commitment to work with them to attain their optimal health. Validation of patient symptoms is the humane and medically responsible way to approach every patient encounter. It is the first step in the process of healing. Patients often walk away from their first visit with me saying that they already feel better. Likewise, when they leave the offices of those who treat them with disdain, their symptoms worsen. Stress plays a huge role in disease and a health care provider can immediately relieve a patient of the stress of being unheard and disbelieved.

Having treated over 900 patients with Morgellons disease since 2003, I have made observations that may be of use to other health care providers. The information that I provide here is intended for physicians, nurse practitioners, physician assistants, naturopaths or other health care providers who are able to prescribe medications.

My suggestions in this chapter are not based upon controlled research studies but rather upon clinical observations with all of the possibilities for uncontrolled variables that this implies. **Patients, please do NOT take the suggestions presented here as a substitute for a visit with your health care provider. None of these medications should be taken without the careful oversight of your provider. Taking treatment into your own hands is a dangerous matter and patients who try this usually do more harm than good.**

Because of the close association of MD with Lyme disease and other tickborne infections, it is imperative to test for these infections using a reputable, specialty lab. I use IGeneX, Inc. Laboratory in Palo Alto, California, 1-800-832-

3200. I have no financial interest in this laboratory. When practitioners read the Lyme Western Blot results they should not pay attention to the "bottom line" of a positive or negative result. Test results are based upon criteria for surveillance, NOT diagnosis. It is important that health care providers be well versed in reading Lyme Western Blots in order to recognize the varying degree of significance of the different bands. An explanation of how to read a Lyme Western Blot is beyond the scope of this book.

Less severe cases of MD have clearing of skin lesions when their underlying infections are treated with the appropriate antibiotics or anti-parasitics. In more severe cases, or cases where no underlying infections are discovered, the addition of an anti-helminthic can be beneficial. To be clear, anthelminthics, commonly known as "de-wormers", are **not** prescribed because we think that a worm causes MD! No research has found any indication of this. Medications often work for purposes other than those for which they were originally intended.

Anthelminthics

Anthelminthics that have been used with success are (in order of most to least effective) ivermectin, albendazole, praziquantel, and mebendazole. Thiabendazole is rarely given due to poor patient tolerability and its having been removed from the commercial market. However, thiabendazole may be compounded and I have had a few cases for which its efficacy has been nothing short of miraculous. The over-the-counter anthelminthic, Pyrantel Pamoate, may be tried but I have rarely seen it be effective.

There are several veterinary anthelminthics that are not available for human use, notably moxidentin and fenbendazole. I have known patients to take these veterinary medications because they are readily available and much less expensive than Rx medications. However, this is

not advisable since they have not been cleared for human use, the dosages are not intended for the size of an average human and they may contain fillers that are harmful or intolerable.

First, Do No Harm

A complete blood count and a comprehensive metabolic panel, which includes liver function tests, are checked monthly and to date, no liver toxicity has been observed and side effects are minimal. Rarely, eosinophilia is seen when patients are on a high dose anthelminthic. This situation resolves when the medication is withdrawn. This tends to happen more frequently with ivermectin than with the others. Unfortunately, ivermectin also seems to be the most effective of them all.

Clinical experience has shown that patients who take probiotics for intestinal health as well as milk thistle and alpha lipoic acid for liver protection have few if any problems. I give a prescription for fluconazole to use as needed for yeast infections. A yeast infection is a signal that the patient is not taking enough probiotics so these should be titrated to individual patient need. *Clostridium difficile* has never been observed except in one case where the patient was NOT taking probiotics as advised. *Saccharomyces boulardii*, a beneficial yeast, is a particularly good probiotic when it comes to avoiding *C.difficile.*

Treatment duration is until resolution of symptoms which can be as little as one year and as long as 6 years. Treatments must be changed frequently due to the apparent adaptability of the pathogen. In some patients, resistance to the treatment method develops as quickly as two weeks. Therefore, frequent follow-ups and treatment changes are necessary.

It is interesting to me that from a clinical standpoint I have not found Lyme disease treatment to be nearly as helpful for MD patients as is the treatment for another tickborne infection,

Bartonellosis. The best approach to the treatment of *Bartonellosis*, and therefore MD, is to give three intracellular antibiotics simultaneously (your prescriber will know what this means) or two intracellular antibiotics and an antiparasitic (like metronidazole, tinidazole, nitazoxanide or atovaquone). I have not found the cell-wall antibiotics (i.e. the penicillins and cephalosporins) to be as effective for MD as they are for Lyme disease. Following are examples of combination therapies that have been successful. I have placed them in order of most effective to least effective. It is best to rotate through these protocols. **Each of these may be given with or without an anti-helminthic.**

Clarithromycin and DS sulfa with or without atovaquone

Doxycycline and rifampin with or without nitazoxanide

Doxycycline and ciprofloxacin with or without tinidazole

Pharmacists usually balk at the quantities of anthelminthics that I prescribe because anthelminthics are usually used for just a few days under normal circumstances. Although I have patients who have taken them daily for many months, I have surprisingly seen no issues with tolerability or toxicity.

When I consider patients psychiatrically and cognitively intact, I will give them prescriptions for the top 3 anthelminthics and instruct them to use just one of them at a time and to change to another when one stops working. Often, 2-week cycles of each seem to work best. (Many patients tell me that they notice that a particular anti-helminthic will cease to be effective after 2 weeks of consecutive use).

Anti-Virals and Antifungals

For a few of my Morgellons patients, the addition of an anti-viral or an anti-fungal has been helpful, so it is always worth giving these each a one-month trial. Again, I believe that when these help it is probably due to lowering a viral or fungal burden from the immune system promoting the enhanced functioning of the patient's natural immunity. I do not think that MD is caused by a virus or a fungus nor do any of the researchers.

Herbal Adjunctive Treatments

1. *BLt Microbial Balancer* by *Researched Nutritionals* can be beneficial. I find it to be helpful in treating *Bartonellosis* and Lyme disease. I usually give this along with antibiotics. *Researched Nutritionals* products need to be purchased through a health care provider who has a contract with the company.

2. Try any of the other herbs that target Bartonella infections such as Sida acuta tincture, Hawthorne tincture, houttuynia powder and EGCg green tea extract. Consult your alternative care practitioner about dosages.

3. I have found that a protocol of 5 different *Beyond Balance* herbal tinctures (listed below) is a good approach for those who will not or cannot take antibiotics. I usually give herbals along *with* antibiotics as I have found in tickborne disease and Morgellons disease that it is a rare patient who does not need both to recover.

My *Beyond Balance* protocol for Morgellons disease consists of the following 5 products, taken together but not simultaneously: MC-BAR 2; TOX-EASE; TOX-EASE GL; PRONAN; and ENL-TX. Each one should be taken separately in about an ounce of water, preferably on an empty stomach. The company supplies dosing instructions. All *Beyond Balance* products are alcohol and gluten-free and need to be purchased through a health care provider who has a contract with the company. I have nothing to gain personally by suggesting any of these products.

General Considerations

In general, there is very high variability to response. What works perfectly for one, won't work at all for another. It is constant trial and error. Patients' feedback is the most important guide to treatment.

Patients need to know that an intensification reaction in early treatment is highly likely. All symptoms, including the skin symptoms of biting and crawling, will worsen before they improve and there is often a mass exodus of fibers. In some patients, the intensification reaction is unbearable requiring medication dosages to be temporarily reduced. Patients need to be aware of this potential reaction and encouraged to "ride it out". Those who do, see results sooner than those who do not.

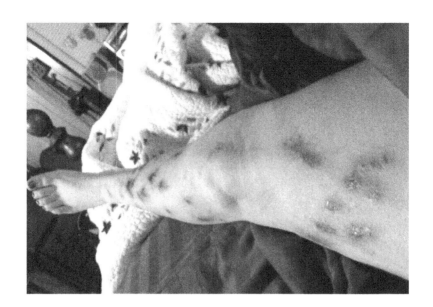

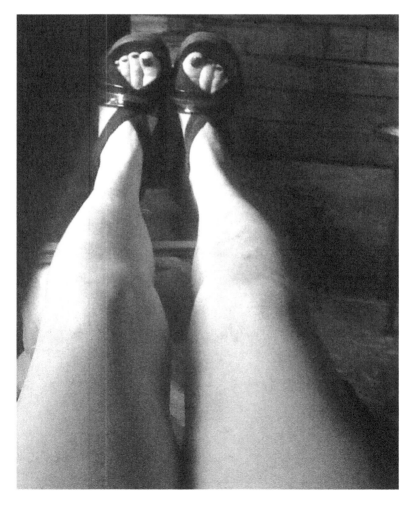

For symptom management, I usually prescribe low dose prescription doxepin at night to help with sleep and itching. The prescription pregabalin has also been helpful for the uncomfortable sensations. It is often beneficial to give an anti-depressant with anti-anxiety properties to help patients cope with the discomforts and stress of the illness. Anti-psychotic medications are not appropriate except in very rare cases. Other suggestions for symptomatic care are listed in the previous chapter.

When patients are compliant, take their medications as directed and maintain regular follow-up appointments, treatment is highly successful. All show improvement and approximately 10% have total resolution of symptoms. I have some patients who have now been off of treatment and symptom-free for five years.

The patients who do not get well are often the ones who are erratic about taking their medications. Unfortunately, there are quite a few of these patients due to the cognitive and psychiatric disabilities inherent in the illness. It is best to involve family members and other loved ones in the patient's care so that they can assist the patient to be compliant.

Any treatment plan must involve uncovering and treating all burdens to the patient's immune status. Strengthening the immune system is at least as important for healing as is giving bactericidal herbs or prescriptions. Examples of possible immune challenges follow. There are entire books written about each of these immune challenges: describing each of the following in detail is beyond the purview of this book.

1. Smoking or exposure to cigarette smoke. Patients must avoid this exposure.

2. Eating inflammatory foods. Patients on an anti-inflammatory diet will improve faster. The first thing that **must** be eliminated is foods containing sugar. For more information see: www.recipesforrepair.com/lyme-inflammation-diet.

3. Mold toxicity. Discover if the patient is currently exposed to mold, remediate the situation or remove the patient from the source and detox. Go to www.survivingmold.com for more information.

4. Occult infection in the sinuses – either bacterial or fungal. Test using www.microbiologydx.com and treat with compounded antibiotic or antifungal nasal sprays.

5. Food allergies. Uncover what they are with the elimination diet and avoid offending foods. Removing gluten from the diet is often helpful for all patients. See www.precisionnutrition.com/elimination-diet

6. Metal toxicity. Testing and treatment by an environmental medicine specialist is necessary.

7. Hypercoagulability or "thick blood". Test and treat.

8. GI problems. SIBO (small intestinal bowel overgrowth), which leads to IBS (irritable bowel syndrome) and leaky gut should be identified and treated. All patients should be on probiotics. Intestinal parasites may be present in those who least expect it. This immune burden should be investigated and treated. Patient should not see a traditional gastrointestinal specialist for this but rather a naturopath or another alternative practitioner who specializes in these issues.

9. Living with high stress. Patients should make every effort possible to remove stressors and when unable to do this should be in therapy to learn to cope.

This chapter has provided a superficial look at the treatment of a very complex disease. Those health care providers interested in knowing more details may email me at

. I cannot provide this information directly to patients so patients should ask their health care providers to email me directly.

Management of Morgellons disease is demanding, so it is not surprising that even those clinicians who believe it to be a physiological illness may not want to accept the challenge of treating it. There is no set protocol to follow, patients are very ill and sometimes have frightening reactions, a tremendous amount of support and availability to the patient is required, and patients' cognitive dysfunction results in non-compliance and dangerous mistakes in following directions. Furthermore, on top of all of the difficulties of actually treating these patients, health care providers have to fear for their licenses due to sanctions by regulatory boards for those treating outside the "standard of care". The fact that there are so few health care providers willing to take on MD patients is not difficult to understand.

FINAL WORDS

The first step in solving the puzzle of Morgellons disease is acceptance of it as a legitimate entity. Health care providers must avoid the temptation to hastily categorize MD patients as delusional, which is happening in medical offices around the world every day. When patients present with unusual symptoms, it is unjust to summarily discount them and relegate them to a psychiatrist's office without a thorough and proper history and exam. If health care providers would take the time and effort to really look at these patients' skin with illuminated magnification they would be amazed and confounded by the unusual things they would see.

The responsibility for a psychiatric diagnosis should not rest in the hands of a primary care provider or a dermatologist. The proper procedure is to refer to a psychiatrist but only after every effort has been made to examine a patient carefully and methodically in order to rule out physiologic abnormalities. The distinguishing characteristic of Morgellons disease is the presence of microscopic subcutaneous filaments, which can be visualized by the examiner with lighted magnification using diligence and patience. The dermatologist must at least make an effort to find the filaments before initiating a psychiatric referral. These filaments are rarely seen without the assistance of magnification.

The diagnosis of a delusional disorder is not one that should be made lightly. Once patients are diagnosed as delusional, the label prejudices other health care providers against them in a never-ending struggle to be taken seriously. A delusional diagnosis can lead to alienation of family and friends and loss of employment. Furthermore, in some cases, children have been removed from the parent with purported DOP. The despair caused by being disregarded leads to isolation and hopelessness and in some cases, suicide.

There are many more "orphan diseases," as they have come to be known, with "orphan" patients abandoned because they did not have the good fortune to come down with a known and socially accepted condition. Throughout the history of medicine we have seen this patient mistreatment due to ignorance on the part of the medical team – patients with tertiary syphilis locked away and put in straight jackets; epileptics believed to be possessed by the devil; gastric ulcer patients advised to learn relaxation techniques because they were inflicting their ailment upon themselves. When patients present with unusual and difficult-to-believe symptoms, health care providers should make sure they are treated with the dignity, attention, and respect that they deserve.

We are David fighting Goliath in this war for the legitimization of Morgellons disease. We

351

are small in numbers but garnering strength from our sense of purpose and righteousness. Our tireless drive is to rescue this group of marginalized patients who do not have the strength nor the influence to stand up for themselves. I agree with the late Swedish neurologist, Dr. Ekbom, and strongly believe that those afflicted with this disease are not and never have been delusional. Their only failing has been in misinterpreting their symptoms and explaining them in a way that does not engender acceptance. In this sense, MD patients have been their own worst enemies. Furthermore, in the few cases where mental illness is involved, it is clearly a consequence rather than a cause of the illness. I would urge that the diagnosis of DOP be abolished from the medical lexicon.

I will end with one last patient story exposing the tragic loss of a sensitive young man with Morgellons disease. May his story impress upon us the urgency of coming to terms with this enigmatic disease.

TRAVIS' STORY

Travis had a way with words. A gentle, timid soul, he was not particularly adept with people but was expressive and insightful in his many writings. He was bright, so much so that despite his young age of 22 he often became impatient with the ineptitude of his fellow humans and the inconsistencies of an irrational world.

Why he developed a mysterious disease that consumed him and made him lose his way is beyond comprehension. "Bug"s, "worms" or things that he couldn't describe seemed to be infesting his body and his brain, tormenting him with itching, biting and stinging sensations. Strange things were occurring that made no sense to his rational mind: fuzz balls, filaments of different colors and black pepper-like dots were emanating from his pores and making his skin feel like it wasn't his own. He couldn't sleep, he couldn't concentrate, he couldn't work or enjoy life in any way. He went from doctor to doctor in desperation, seeking to discover the cause of his misery, hoping to find a diagnosis to explain his bizarre symptoms. He hoped that even if none could diagnose his malady, someone might at least listen, look, and try to understand and help him.

Hope slipped away with each succeeding office visit. He appeared pale, thin, anxious, fearful and covered with open sores. Immediate diagnoses of "delusions of parasitosis", "self-mutilation" or "methamphetamine abuse" were conferred upon him without a proper history or physical. Health care providers would shake their heads in judgmental haste and refer him on to a psychiatrist.

Was he crazy? It sure seemed that way. But his craziness didn't cause the illness. The illness caused the craziness. He became obsessed with every little detail of his hygiene and of his surroundings. He tirelessly scrutinized every inch of his body, looking for signs of his invader and hoping to extract the instruments of his torture. He felt terribly sick emotionally and physically. He had to drop out of school and quit his job as a pharmacy technician. The lesions that covered his body were an eyesore. He was embarrassed to be seen in public for fear that others would think he was contagious or unclean. For over a year he stayed locked up in his room, hiding from the world, unable to live a normal life or look forward to a promising future. His only connections to the outside world were the web blog that he faithfully maintained and the chat groups he was a part of.

This is an excerpt from one of many emails that Travis sent me during this time:

"Since I've had this disease, I've never laughed, I've never felt content or happy and I've never had a good time. I always think of suicide when I have Morgellons attacks because of the highly traumatic nature of them. They make me want to jump out of my skin and just make me feel

like I'm in Hell. I've stared into the abyss for so long that it's not just staring back at me anymore; we've become one single entity. So I've said goodbye to the idea of me ever being able to use my Super-ego or even my Ego. I have become my Id. [In Freudian psychology the Id is the primitive and instinctive component of personality with survival and fulfillment of basic needs the driving forces. The personality of a newborn baby is all "Id"].

The turning point for Travis came when he read an article that I wrote about the "mysterious skin condition known as Morgellons disease". As he read, he gasped as he recognized every one of his symptoms. For the first time in several years, he felt a glimmer of hope. Finally, someone would take him seriously and would treat him with respect. He came to see me and after a thorough history and exam I informed him that he fit the criteria for this unusual and little-known disease, a disease for which there was no test or cure, a disease that, although described over 300 years before, was not even recognized by the Centers for Disease Control and Prevention (CDC) or state health departments.

Validation of his illness was a huge step but there were more obstacles to overcome. I explained to Travis that since the causative agent of MD has yet to be discovered, its treatment is a shot in the dark. The patient must surrender himself as lab rat, willingly taking different concoctions of antibiotics that have been helpful to others with the same affliction, but never knowing whether he will be one of the lucky ones who respond. I explained that some patients with MD, especially those with long-standing illness, have worsening symptoms with treatment. Their condition becomes aggravated and their sensitivities sharpened. Anxiety peaks, discomfort heightens and the unusual objects flow forth with a vengeance.

This was the case with Travis. His response to treatment was such an intensification of symptoms that on several occasions his mother took him to the local psychiatric hospital, not knowing how to handle his agitation and his inability to cope with the pain. If he then stopped treatment his manic episodes would disappear but the return to baseline was a return to the same lonely life of despair. From past experience, I knew that our only hope was to treat with antibiotics, but his reaction to treatment was insupportable so it was difficult to know how to proceed. I believed that his case was too complex for me to handle, but there were no doctors in the entire country that would know what to do or even take his disease seriously.

We seemed to be caught between a rock and a hard place. We'd take one step forward and two steps back. Meanwhile, other MD patients of mine were having symptom flares but getting past them and going on to notice a marked improvement with antibiotics. But without improvement, there was no hope. Eventually, life with pain and fear and without dignity or hope seemed pointless and unbearable.

One Sunday afternoon the horror of it all became too much for Travis to bear. In search of sleep and pain relief he took what proved to be an excess of sedating medications and slipped away from his earthly prison. His mother found him a few hours later and through the shock and sorrow, she couldn't help but notice that it was the first time in several years she had seen a peaceful look on his face. A strange mix of feelings overcame her – the gut-wrenching agony of a mother losing her only precious son mixed with a sense of relief that his suffering was finally over.

What happened to Travis should make everyone in the medical field pause and consider the ways that they treat patients. Patients deserve to be listened to and taken seriously. To confer a hasty psychiatric diagnosis when a patient's symptoms seem too unusual to categorize is as much a transgression against humanity as it is medical malpractice. Since Travis' untimely death, other MD patients have died under similar circumstances – desperately trying to find relief from suffering to the point of overdose, often by accident and undoubtedly, at times, on purpose.

Soon before he died Travis sent me the following email. His words are a sad testament to modern health care. Patient advocacy should be at the top of every health care provider's priority list.

"Most doctors seem cold and distant and treat patients like something other than human beings. The doctor that I saw in the ER who diagnosed me with Delusional Parasitosis comes to mind the most since he only talked to me for about 2 minutes, refused to examine me, and did not care in the slightest about whether I was doing alright or not. You made me realize that passion for patients' health is not a lost art and this gives me hope".

The tragedy of young Travis' life and death should serve as an admonition to health care providers not to abandon a patient by disregarding his concerns, ignoring his feelings, or discounting his suffering. That is not the way that anyone would want to be treated nor would anyone tolerate that kind of disrespect for someone they love. Unfortunately, there are tens of thousands more like Travis. Let us not forsake them; let us devote our time and resources to researching this horrific disease so that others may be spared its devastating effects.

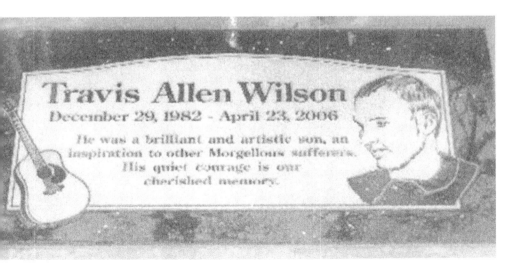

GLOSSARY OF TERMS
AND ACRONYMS

Alginate - aka Alginic Acid, is a sugar and a gelling substance.

ALS - Amyotrophic Lateral Sclerosis, aka Lou Gehrig's disease, is a type of motor neuron disease involving the death of nerve cells that control muscular movement.

Anthelminthic - A type of medication used in the treatment of intestinal worms or nematodes.

Atrophy - v. To waste away.

Autoimmune disease - A disease in which the body's immune cells attack the body's own healthy cells.

Bb - Abbreviation for *Borrelia burgdorferi,* the spiral-shaped bacteria that cause Lyme disease.

Biofilm - A protective colony of bacteria, stuck together with a slimy substance.

Biopsy - Removal of live tissue from the body to be examined under microscopy.

Bradykinin – An inflammatory peptide that causes blood vessels to dilate and consequently blood pressure to fall.

CEHMDF - The Charles E. Holman Morgellons Disease Foundation.

Collagen - The most abundant protein in the human body and the main component of connective tissue. It basically holds the body together.

Delusion - A fixed belief in something that cannot be supported by evidence or logic. Delusions can be visual, auditory or tactile.

Dermatoscope – Magnification tool used by doctors to closely examine the skin.

DOP - Delusions of Parasitosis – the false belief that one is infected with parasites.

DSM-5 - Fifth edition (2013) of the Diagnostic and Statistical Manual of Mental Disorders.

Electron microscopy – A microscope capable of high resolution and high magnification allowing visualization of very small objects in fine detail.

Electrostatic charge - An excess or deficiency of electrons, causing close objects to be drawn together or repelled from one another.

Eosinophilia - An excess of eosinphils, a type of white blood cells. Often signals an allergic reaction or an infection with parasites.

Epidemiology - The study of diseases from the standpoint of distribution, incidence, prevalence and geography.

Epidermis - The outer layer of skin.

Etiology - The cause of a disease.

EBP - Evidenced based practice.

Fibroblasts - Cells that specialize in producing collagen and other fibers.

Formication - The sensation that insects are crawling all over the skin.

Fungal infection - Infections caused by a fungus or yeast such as athlete's foot or systemic candidiasis.

GMO - Genetically modified organism. A laboratory process where the gene of one species is transferred into an unrelated species.

Hair follicle - The covering around the root of a hair.

Hypochondriac - A person who suffers from anxiety about their health and worries about every little symptom believing it to be something serious.

Immunosuppressive therapy - Treatment with medications that quiet the immune response, particularly used in cases where this is necessary such as organ transplants and autoimmune diseases.

Indolent infection - An infection that is low-grade or slow to develop.

Jarish-Herxheimer Reaction - A worsening of symptoms that occurs about 4 to 5 days into antibiotic treatment of spirochetal infections.

Keratin - A protein that is the main structural component of hair, nails and the outer layer of the skin.

Keratinocyte - A skin cell that produces keratin.

Lyme disease - An infection caused by the spriochetal bacteria *Borrelia burgdorferi,* usually acquired through the bite of a tick. Lyme disease can affect every body system, causing many and varied symptoms.

MD - Morgellons disease (medical doctor = M.D.).

Melanin - The pigment that gives skin, hair and eyes their coloration. The more melanin in the tissue, the darker the color.

MRF - Morgellons Research Foundation (now defunct).

Neurodegenerative diseases - A group of diseases resulting from the deterioration or death of nerve cells.

Neuropathy - Disease of peripheral nerves leading to weakness, numbness, tingling and pain.

OSU - Oklahoma State University.

Parasite - An organism that depends on another organism in order to stay alive.

Pathogenic - Any organism that can cause disease.

PPI - Proton pump inhibitor, a medication that shuts down acid production in the stomach.

Proliferation - Growth, leading to increase in numbers.

Pruritis - Severe itching of the skin.

Punch biopsy - A type of small, circular skin biopsy which is deep enough to include the full thickness of the skin.

Spirochete – A microscopic, spiral-shaped bacterium.

Ultraviolet (UV) light - aka "black light".

Western Blot - A type of blood test that looks for specific antibodies to an organism.

BIBLIOGRAPHY

Ahn C, Mulligan P, Salcido RS (2008). Smoking, the
    bane of wound healing; Biomedical
    interventions and social influences.
    Advances in Skin and Wound Care, 21(5),
    237 – 238.

Bernard P (2008). Management of common
    bacterial infections of the skin. *Current
    Opinion in Infectious Diseases, 21*(2), 122-
    128.

Ekbom, KA (2003). The Pre-senile Delusion of
    Infestation in *History of Psychiatry*, 14:232.
    New York: Sage Publications.

Evans NJ, Brown JM, Demirkan I, et al. Association
    of unique, isolated treponemes with
    bovine digital dermatitis lesions. *J Clin
    Microbiol*. 2009;47:689–696.

Frieman A, Bird G, Metelitsa AI, Barankin B, Lauzon
    GJ (2004).Cutaneous effects of smoking.
    *Journal of Cutaneous Medicine and Surgery:
    Incorporating Medical and Surgical
    Dermatology, 8*(6), 415-423.

Georgilis K, Peacocke M, Klempner MS (1992).
    Fibroblasts protect the Lyme disease

spirochete, Borrelia burgdorferi, from ceftriaxone in vitro. *Journal of Infectious Diseases,* 8;166(2), 440-4.

Glieck, James. *Chaos: Making a New Science.* Open Road Media, 2011.

Gomez A, Cook NB, Bernardoni ND, et al. An experimental model to induce digital dermatitis infection in cattle. *J Dairy Sci* 2012;95(4):1821-1830/

Gordin MD. *The Pseudoscience Wars.* University of Chicago Press, 2012.

Harvey WT (2007). Morgellons disease. *Journal of the American Academy of Dermatology, 56,* 705-706.308). Amsterdam: Ios Press.

Institute of Medicine Committee on Quality of Health Care in America (2001). *Crossing the Quality Chasm: A New Health System for the 21st Century.* Washington, DC: National Academies Press.

Kellett CE (1935). Sir Thomas Browne and the disease called the Morgellons. *Annals of Medical History, 7,* 467-469.

Klempner MS, Rogers RA, Noring R (1993). Invasion of fibroblasts by the Lyme spirochete *Borrelia burgdorferi*. J Infect Dis. 167:1074–1081.

Koblenzer CS (2006). The challenge of Morgellons disease. *Journal of the American Academy of Dermatology. 55*, 920-922.

Koo J, Gambla C (1996). Cutaneous sensory disorder. *Dermatology Clinics, 14*(3), 497-502.

Kuruvlia M, Gahalaut P, Zacharia A (2004). A study of skin disorders in patients with primary psychiatric conditions. *Indian Journal of Dermatology, Venereology, and Leprology, 70*(5), 292-295.

Lee MR & Shumack S (2005). Prurigo nodularis: A review. *Australasian Journal of Dermatology. 46*(4): 211-220.

Lutfi A (2016). Ekbom Syndrome, an evidenced based review of literature. *Asian Journal of Medical Sciences*, 7(3), 1-7.

Markle WH & Makhoul K (2004). Cutaneous leishmaniasis: Recognition and treatment. *American Family Physician, 69*(6), 1455-1460.

Mayne P, English JS, Kilbane EJ, Burke JM, Middelveen MJ, Stricker RB. Morgellons: a novel dermatological perspective as the multisystem infective disease borreliosis. *F1000 Res.* 2013;2:118.

Mehta RK, Burrows NP, Payne CM, Mendelsohn SS, Pope FM, Rytina E (2001). Elastosis perforans serpiginosa and associated disorders. *Clinical and Experimental Dermatology, 26*, 521-524.

Middelveen MJ, Bandoski C, Burke J, Sapi E, Filush KR, Wang Y, Franco A, Mayne PJ, Stricker RB. (2015) Exploring the association between Morgellons disease and Lyme disease: identification of *Borrelia burgdorferi* in Morgellons disease patients. *BMC Dermatol.* 5(1):1.

Middelveen MJ, Burugu D, Poruri A, Burke J, Mayne PJ, Sapi E, et al. Association of spirochetal infection with Morgellons disease. *F1000 Res.* 2013;2:25.

Middelveen MJ, Mayne PJ, Kahn DG, Stricker RB. Characterization and evolution of dermal filaments from patients with Morgellons disease. *Clin Cosmet Investig Dermatol.* 2013;6:1–21.

Middelveen MJ, Poruri A, Mayne PJ, Sapi E, Kahn DG, Stricker RB. Association of *Borrelia burgdorferi* infection with Morgellons disease. *J Invest Med.* 2013;61:225.

Middelveen MJ, Rasmussen EH, Kahn DG, Stricker RB. Morgellons disease: A chemical and light microscopic study. J Clin Exp Dermatol Res. 2012;3:140.

Middelveen MJ, Stricker RB. Filament formation associated with spirochetal infection: A comparative approach to Morgellons disease. *Clin Cosmet Investig Dermatol.* 2011;4:167–177.

Middelveen MJ, Stricker RB. Morgellons disease: a filamentous borrelial dermatitis. *Int Journal of General Medicine,* 2016:9.

Mills CM (1998). Cigarette smoking, cutaneous immunity, and inflammatory response. *Clinics in Dermatology, 16,* 589 – 594.

O'Donnell, M. A sceptic's medical dictionary. London: BMJ Books, 1997.

Polat M, Oztas P, Ilhan M, Yalcin B, Alli N (2008). Generalized pruritis: A prospective study concerning etiology. *American Journal of Clinical Dermatology, 9*(1), 39-44.

Rapini RP, Herbert AA, Drucker CR (1989). Acquired perforating dermatoses: Evidence for combined transepidermal elimination of both collagen and elastic fibers. *Archives of Dermatology*, *125*, 1074-1078.

Savely V, Kennedy B, Ernst E (2010). Morgellons Disease in a 48 Year-old Female with Dermatologic Complaints, *Advanced Emergency Nursing Journal*, 32(4); 314-322.

Savely G, Leitao MM (2005). Skin lesions and crawling sensation: disease or delusion? *Adv Nurse Pract*. 13:16–17.

Savely V. (2010) Delusions May not always be Delusions. *Arch Psychiatr Nurs*, 24(4): 215.

Savely VR, Leitao MM, Stricker RB (2006). The mystery of Morgellons disease: Infection or delusion? *Am J Clin Dermatol*. 7:1–5.

Savely VR, Stricker RB (2007). Morgellons disease: the mystery unfolds. *Expert Rev Dermatol*. 2:585–591.

Savely VR, Stricker RB (2010). Morgellons disease: analysis of a population with clinically confirmed microscopic subcutaneous fibers of unknown etiology. *Clin Cosmet Investig Dermatol.* 3:67–78.

Segarra-Newnham M (2007). Manifestations, diagnosis, and treatment of *Strongyloides stercoralis* infection. *The Annals of Pharmacotherapy, 41*(12), 1992 – 2001.

Sehgal VN, Jain S, Thappa DM, Bhattacharya SN, Logani K (1993). Perforating dermatoses: a review and report of four cases. *Journal of Dermatology. 20*, 329-340.

Stander S, Schmetz M (2006). Chronic itch and pain: Similarities and differences. *European Journal of Pain, 10*(5), 473-478.

Stander S, Steinhoff M, Schmetz M, Weisshaar E, Metze D, Luger T (2003). Neurophysiology of Pruritus. *Archives of Dermatology, 139*(11), 1463-1470.

Stander S, Weisshaer E, Mettang T, Szepietowski JC, Carstens E, Ikoma A et al (2007). Clinical classification of itch: A position paper of the International Forum for the Study of Itch. *Acta Dermato- Venereol*ogica, *87*(4), 291-294.

Stricker RB, Middelveen MJ (2012). Morgellons disease: More questions than answers. *Psychosomatics.* 53(5):504–505.

Stricker RB, Savely VR, Motanya NC, Giglas BC (2009). Complement split products C3a and C4a in chronic Lyme disease. *Scandinavian Journal of Immunology, 69*(1), 64-69.

Stricker RB, Savely VR, Zaltsman A, Citovsky V (2007). Contribution of *Agrobacterium* to Morgellons disease. *Journal of Investigative Medicine. 55*, S123.

Stricker RB, Winger EE (2001). Decreased CD57 lymphocyte subset in patients with chronic Lyme disease. *Immunological Letters, 76*(1), 43-48.

Ude S, Arnold DL, Moon CD, Timms-Wilson T, Spiers AJ (2006). Biofilm formation and cellulose expression among diverse environmental *Pseudomonas* isolates. *Environmental Microbiology, 8*, 1997-2011.

Wood S, Data A, Pabbat N, Burugu P, Ratelle A (2015). Differentiation of Borrelia microbes from collagen debris and collagen fibrils in blood cultures. *Journal of Microbiology and Experimentation, 2*(1).

Wymore RS, Casey RL, Allen RW, Boese M, Pogue R, Burkeen J. Physical evidence in Morgellons disease. Presented at the 14th International Molecular Medicine Tri-Conference, San Francisco, CA, February 27-March 2, 2007.

Zirwas MJ & Seraly MP (2001). Pruritus of unknown origin: A retrospective study. *Journal of the American Academy of Dermatology, 45*(6), 892-896.

ACKNOWLEDGEMENTS

Rob Hutchins, my loving husband. Thank you for your patience and for your excellent proof reading and feedback.

Cindy Casey, my steadfast companion in the struggle for Morgellons disease recognition. Your dedication and compassion are beyond compare and your wise counsel led me through this process. Thank you for your logical thinking and your sense of humor!

Chas Holman, gone but never-to-be forgotten. He was the first non-medical person who did not have the disease himself to devote his life to advocating for the recognition of Morgellons disease.

Bill Harvey, may he rest in peace, who was the first medical doctor to take Morgellons disease seriously and collaborate with me on how to help its sufferers.

And for their invaluable assistance in various ways (in alphabetical order): Harriet Bishop, Bob Bransfield, Nancy Egger, Ruben de Haas, Deborah Markel, Marianne Middelveen, Denise Moudree, Carsten Nicolaus, Elizabeth and Edward Rasmussin, Eva Sapi, Jyotsna Shah, Gwen Simmons, Ray Stricker, Michael Ulmschneider, Randy Wymore and Lisa Von Behren.

ABOUT THE AUTHOR

Virginia "Ginger" Savely grew up in Annapolis, Maryland and received her first Bachelor's degrees in Psychology and Music from the University of Maryland in 1972. After a 13-year career as a singer/songwriter/performer she went back to school at the University of Texas at Austin and became a nurse in 1988 and a family nurse practitioner in 1998. She earned her doctorate degree in 2008 from Case Western Reserve University where she conducted research on Morgellons disease.

Ginger started out in primary care and began to identify so many Lyme patients in her practice that she gradually became a Lyme specialist. She has been treating and advocating for Morgellons disease since 2003. Ginger has received many awards recognizing her prowess as a health care provider. Her practice, TBD Medical Associates, located previously in Austin, TX and San Francisco, CA is currently in Washington, DC. Her patients come to her from all over the US and several other countries.

As of June 2015, Ginger and her husband live most of the year in San Miguel de Allende, Mexico. She still maintains an office in Washington, DC where she goes every few months to see patients and visit her family, including 2 grandchildren. Ginger travels all over the US and Europe giving presentations on Lyme and other tickborne diseases as well as Morgellons disease. She is on the medical advisory board of the CEHMDF and has published numerous journal and magazine articles. This is her first book.

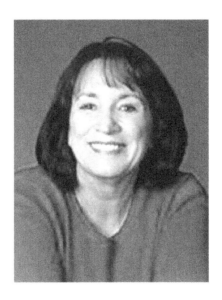

For more information on Morgellons Disease,
please visit www.morgellonsdisease.org

To access color versions of the photographs
contained in this book, please visit
www.gingersavely.com/morgellons-book